CW00801554

LymphoedemaUnited

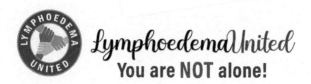

You are NOT alone!

LymphoedemaUnited

You are NOT alone!

Lymphoedema stories from around the world
Volume 1

Lymphoedema affects millions of people around the world, yet it is often a lottery whether the appropriate level of healthcare is received. That can leave a person living with this lifelong disease feeling desperate, neglected, and alone.

You are NOT alone!

Advocates Amy Rivera and Matt Hazledine are joined by 34 people living with lymphoedema from 14 countries from around the world, who share their personal experiences and top tips, to help you to live better with lymphoedema.

COMPILED BY
**AMY RIVERA &
MATT HAZLEDINE**

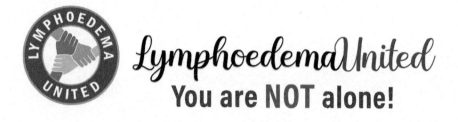

First published 2023 by Wordzworth Publishing

ISBN: 978-1-78324-287-0 (paperback)
ISBN: MISSING (ebook)

Book design and typesetting by *www.wordzworth.com*

Dedicated to everyone living with lymphoedema, a lifelong and sometimes debilitating disease that is challenging both physically and mentally. You are NOT alone!

Thank you to all our guests, who have written openly and honestly about their journey and experiences of living with lymphoedema. Our collective aim is to promote unity within the lymphoedema community and help others living with this chronic condition.

We are very grateful to be supported by Sigvaris Group, medi and Juzo. Jobst is also featured in the book. Thank you.

CONTENTS

FOREWORD

Professor Christine Moffatt CBE
Chair of the International Lymphoedema Framework

It is a great privilege and honour to be asked to write the forward to this important book that portrays the reality of people living with Lymphoedema throughout the world and the courage that is described in their stories. I am currently the chair of a charity the International Lymphoedema Framework (ILF) and I established this work because of the desperate plight affecting millions of people living with Lymphoedema worldwide and the lack of awareness and effective treatment in many countries.

Lymphoedema is truly a worldwide problem that has very many different causes, yet despite this we do not have accurate information about how many people are suffering and, in many countries; there are little or no services available. I think of Lymphoedema as a ***hidden neglected global*** condition that has been ignored despite the terrible burden on people and their families. Charities such as the ILF are trying to bring everyone together to solve these issues and believe that patients are the central reason why this is needed.

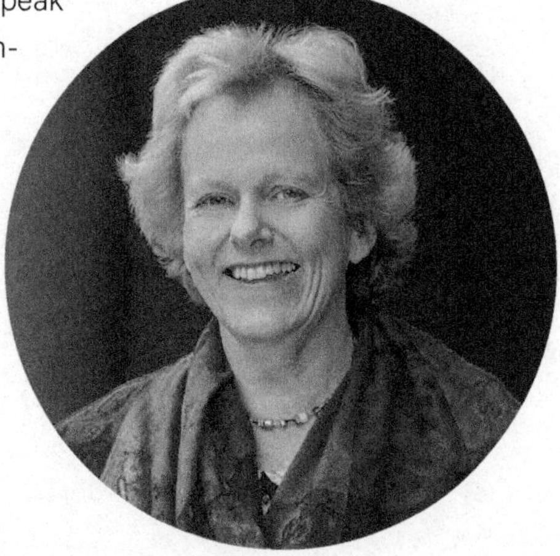

The stories in this wonderful book speak of the emotional impact of the condition but they also show us the power of emotional resilience from these individuals who have fought to take a level of control over their condition and to obtain treatment. In my research with children and families coping with Lymphoedema a similar story emerges and it speaks of isolation, despair, and loneliness.

But I want to bring you a message of hope that the professional world is waking up to these issues and we have over the last 10 years seen great strides in diagnosis and treatment. My heart goes out to you all because I know that what you long for is to be cured. While this is not possible yet, nevertheless the knowledge that is being gained from genetic studies is beginning to unravel the conundrum and offers tangible hope for treatments and possible cure in the future.

If you are reading this book and asking yourself well how does this help me today? I ask you to gain courage from the stories which show how people living with Lymphoedema have learnt to manage their condition and I encourage you to join the Lymphoedema patient organisations that exist. It is other people who suffer with the condition who have that true and deep understanding and provide invaluable support and tips for day-to day-life.

This book is written by people living with Lymphoedema and donations made from the profits will be given to those who need help. The ILF have been asked to help this initiative, and we are so delighted to do so. The motto for the ILF is ***belonging together*** and I can promise you that this community will continue to strive to obtain care for people across the world. We will lobby at every level from the World Health Organisation, healthcare systems and professional bodies and we will always ensure that people living with Lymphoedema are at the heart of every initiative.

Please do not give up hope. With effective treatment this condition can be controlled, and you are not alone in your journey.

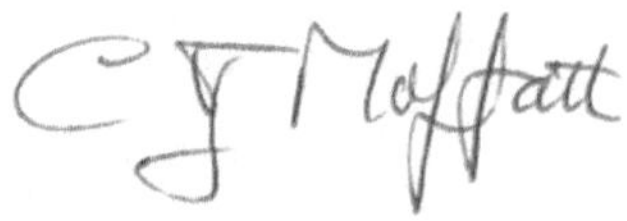

PREFACE

WHERE DID THE IDEA FOR THIS BOOK COME FROM?

Completely coincidentally on 1st October 2021, both Matt Hazledine and Amy Rivera launched their very first books, each sharing their personal journey living with lymphoedema, or lymphedema depending on where you are from.

Matt's book 'How to live better with lymphoedema – Meet the Experts' documented his ten years of experiences and tips, alongside over 20 lymphoedema experts writing trusted information and valuable guidance.

Amy's book 'Drop the Skirt' tells her story from her earliest memories of living with lymphedema, since birth, hiding it throughout her teenage years until she was inspired to change her mindset and unknowingly, at the time, her life.

Matt created a patient-based website called lymphoedemaunited.com, which includes a section called 'Meet the Members', where others with lymphoedema share their story and challenges, some include their social media addresses to invite others to unite with them.

After a few online meetings, Matt and Amy decided to collaborate on turning this concept into a book and started inviting people they knew to discuss this project. Almost everyone they approached, from many parts of the world, agreed to participate and the concept soon became a reality.

Our aim is for this to be the first volume of many to unite the lymphoedema community. If you are interested in sharing your story in future editions, please email *matt@lymphunited.com* or *amy@winourfight.org*

We hope you find this book both helpful and inspiring.

Matt Hazledine & Amy Rivera

MEDICAL ADVICE DISCLAIMER

DISCLAIMER: THIS BOOK DOES NOT PROVIDE MEDICAL ADVICE

All material in this book is for informational purposes only and is not a substitute for professional medical advice, diagnosis, or treatment.

Always seek the advice of your physician or other qualified healthcare provider with any questions you may have regarding a medical condition or treatment and before undertaking a new health care regime. Never disregard professional medical advice or delay in seeking it because of something you have read in this book.

Reliance on any information provided in this book by the authors/compilers and others featured in the book is solely at your own risk.

Any information and guidance written in this book by any medical expert, organisation, company, or guest has not been changed by the authors/compliers. Content written by the authors/compilers, is done so in the context of providing insights as people living with lymphoedema and should not be considered as medical advice in any capacity.

For the avoidance of any doubt, Matt Hazledine and Amy Rivera both have lymphoedema and they are not medical professionals.

Product & Services Disclaimer

The information, products, and services mentioned in this book are provided for informational purposes only. While we strive to provide accurate and up-to-date information, we do not assume any responsibility or liability for the use or misuse of any products or services mentioned. Readers are encouraged to conduct their own research and exercise their own judgment when considering the use or purchase of any products or services. The views and opinions expressed in this book are those of the authors and do not necessarily reflect our own views or opinions.

Authenticity of Content

It is important to note that any content written by our guests has not been changed and therefore, we do not take any responsibility for the accuracy of the information provided.

To ensure that the book is authentic and honest, all content written by Matt and Amy has not been edited by an expert ghost writer or a publisher.

All prices quoted in the book are in GBP and correct at the time of going to print.

1

INTRODUCTION

By Matt Hazledine

If you are reading this, the chances are that you either have lymphoedema (lymphedema), know someone that does, or work in the medical profession caring for people with this lifelong and sometimes debilitating disease.

The Lymphatic Education & Research Network (LE&RN) estimates that hundreds of millions of people worldwide, suffer from lymphoedema and lymphatic diseases. LE&RN state on their website, that more people suffer from these diseases in the USA than suffer from Multiple Sclerosis, Muscular Dystrophy, ALS, Parkinson's disease and AIDS combined, which is staggering.

Yet, many of us experience a varying level of professional care from medical experts IF you have been successful in getting a diagnosis. Many are still seeking a diagnosis, which means that they are unlikely to be receiving the appropriate health care and advice on self-management techniques, which is important during the early stages of lymphoedema.

This can result in people feeling helpless, alone and desperate. Lymphoedema can be extremely challenging to both physical and mental health, especially when coming to terms with the diagnosis and adapting to this life-changing condition.

Some people are willing to talk about their health issue, while others keep it hidden. Some people confidently wear their compression garments in public, while others hide it under baggy clothes and some people just don't or can't go out at all.

You are NOT alone!

This book includes personal experiences and tips from 34 people from 14 different countries. Some have primary and some have secondary lymphoedema, effecting their arms, legs, trunk, head, neck, and pubic area. They were willing to share their story to reassure others they are not alone. Some guests have included their contact details, so, if you relate to their circumstances, you can connect with them directly.

Our other aim is to support lymphoedema charities around the world, by donating a proportion of the annual pre-tax profits from this book, which we hope will continue for many years to come.

Thank you for purchasing our book. We hope you find it helpful. If so, please recommend it to others living with lymphoedema.

Matt Hazledine

By Amy Rivera

Welcome to "Lymphedema United: You Are Not Alone," an extraordinary anthology that weaves together the diverse stories of individuals from all corners of the world who have embarked on a courageous journey with lymphedema. Within these pages, you will discover a powerful collection of personal narratives that illuminate the triumphs, challenges, and remarkable resilience of those living with this condition.

At its core, this anthology celebrates the power of storytelling. It is through the art of sharing our experiences, our triumphs, and even our vulnerabilities that we forge deep connections and foster a sense of community. As we unite our voices, we create a harmonious chorus, echoing the message that no one with lymphedema should ever feel isolated or alone.

Through these heartfelt stories, we aim to spread awareness about lymphedema, shedding light on the complexities and realities of living with this often-misunderstood condition. Each unique journey unfolds with honesty, compassion, and authenticity, giving voice to the diverse perspectives and lived experiences of individuals who have faced the trials and tribulations associated with lymphedema head-on.

But this anthology is more than a collection of personal narratives; it is a platform for change and empowerment. By embracing the power of storytelling, we seek to redefine the narrative surrounding lymphedema, shifting the focus from limitations to possibilities, from despair to hope, and from isolation to community. It is our collective mission to promote a positive view of living with lymphedema, inspiring others to embrace their journey with strength, resilience, and unwavering determination.

You will discover stories of personal growth, medical breakthroughs, and the indomitable human spirit. You will witness the transformative power of self-acceptance and the profound impact of finding support and understanding from others who have walked a similar path. From the challenges of diagnosis to the triumphs of managing symptoms, these stories resonate with authenticity and offer valuable insights into navigating the complexities of living with lymphedema.

As you dive into the depths of these narratives, prepare to be moved, enlightened, and inspired. You will witness the unwavering spirit of individuals who refuse to let lymphedema define them, who embrace their uniqueness, and who find strength in the face of adversity. These stories remind us that even in the darkest moments, there is always light to guide us forward.

"Lymphedema United: You Are Not Alone" is an embodiment of the global lymphedema community. It transcends borders, cultures, and languages to remind us that we are united by our shared experiences and our unwavering determination to live life to the fullest. It serves as a testament to the power of community and the remarkable strength that emerges when we stand together, shoulder to shoulder.

So, embark on this transformative journey with an open heart and an open mind. Allow the stories within this anthology to touch your soul, ignite your compassion, and instil within you a sense of profound understanding. May the power of storytelling guide us toward a world where awareness thrives, where support abounds, and where no one with lymphedema ever feels alone.

Welcome to "Lymphedema United: You Are Not Alone."

Amy Rivera

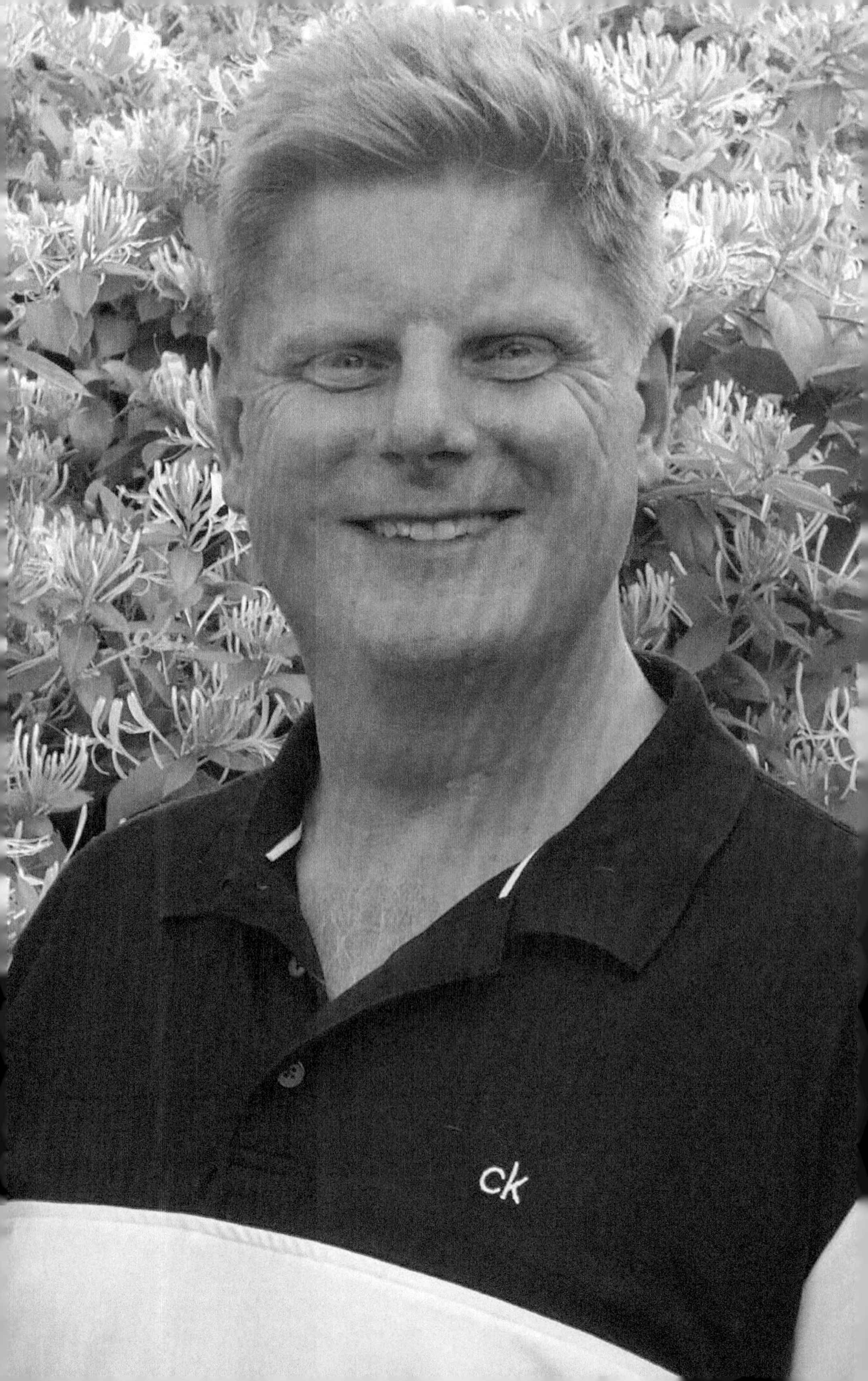
ck

2

MATT HAZLEDINE

> ***Cellulitis is the most painful thing I've experienced, which could've led to the amputation of my leg.***

The day my life changed forever was Saturday 18th June 2011, the day before Father's Day. After returning home from a shopping trip with my wife and daughter for my gift, I became ill, quite suddenly, with strong flu-like symptoms including a fever and convulsions. It was unlike anything I'd experienced before, and it was quite scary, especially when my temperature reached over 40°C. Apparently, by this point, I was a bit delirious, and my wife was concerned enough to take me to hospital.

We arrived in Accident & Emergency (A&E) and it wasn't long before I was moved to a side room and given intravenous morphine to help control the pain. Within a couple of hours, I was admitted to a ward and put under observation. The initial diagnosis was a skin infection, and I was prescribed intravenous antibiotics, which took several hours to be administered.

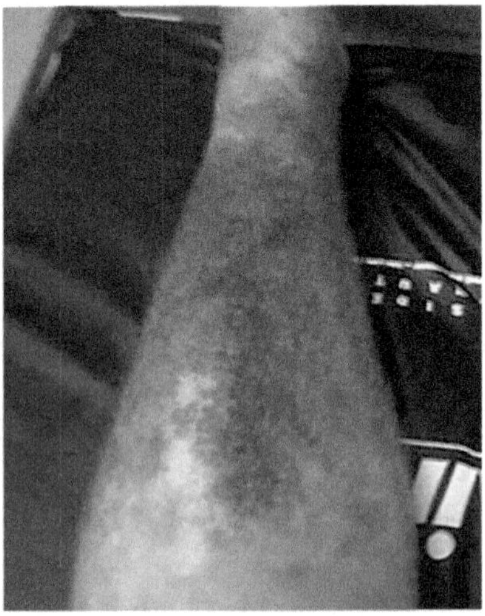

Matt Hazledine - Cellulitis in left leg, June 2011

I soon became aware of a small red rash on my left shin, about the size of a 5p piece. It was hot and itchy and became very painful. It was frightening to watch it spread incredibly rapidly, covering my complete lower leg before moving to my thigh, literally within a few hours of being admitted. I had never seen anything like it before and never experienced such excruciating pain. When standing to visit the bathroom, the pain was so intense that I had to use a walking frame and shuffle. It felt as though acid was being poured down my leg. A pain I will never forget to this day. After a couple of days, the rash became even more widespread and painful and I was sent for several tests, including an X-ray to rule out necrotising fasciitis. A positive diagnosis could lead to amputation of my leg. My mind was spinning with the 'what-if' scenarios; I was 40 with two young daughters and had started a new business venture 6-months before. Thankfully, it wasn't the flesh-eating disease and amputation wasn't required.

Later that day, the blood cultures showed that there were Staphylococcus and Streptococcus bacteria present, and I was diagnosed with an infection called cellulitis. It appeared that the bacteria may have entered via an open blister on my little toe. With the infection correctly identified, I was immediately put on a cocktail of intravenous and oral antibiotics, with a side order of painkillers including the odd hit of Oramorph when the pain was at its peak. Despite the doctor confirming that the combination of antibiotics was equivalent to 'bleach', it took five days for my temperature to come down.

I spent 13 nights and 14 long days in hospital, cared for by some wonderful nurses. During my second week, my leg started to swell, quite noticeably, from foot to thigh, which raised much concern. None of the medical staff seemed to know why or what it was. Later that week I was visited by a Consultant Vascular Surgeon, who told me, very bluntly, that I now had a lifelong disease called lymphoedema. I was told to see the Supplies Team for a stocking before being discharged. And that was that. The total extent of the explanation that I received. A stocking? What is this disease? What is the treatment? How long would my leg be swollen for? Where do I go for help? I received nothing, nada, nichts, rien, absolutely nowt!

I was given two off-the-shelf circular knit stockings from the Supplies Team. I enquired about receiving further garments and received a huge sigh followed by 'you'll have to ask your GP.' That was the magnitude of the aftercare at that early stage of diagnosis. I left hospital on day 14 about to face the unknown, feeling abandoned, scared, and desperate.

Lymphoedema is a disease that is with me for life. The first few years after diagnosis were incredibly difficult for me and my family, and in fact my lowest point ever. The numerous challenges affected me physically and mentally. We searched for information, help and solutions which took too long to find, during which my leg was increasing in size. The off-the-shelf basic stocking was totally wrong for me and insufficient to contain the swelling. It was a challenging period of my life, affecting my morale and self-confidence, home life, work life and relationships. I couldn't fit into any of my suit trousers, jeans, or shoes. I now know that I am not the only one who went through this period of despair, although at the time it was the loneliest place in the world. Men don't tend to talk about their health and feelings, and I had fallen into that trap. More about that later.

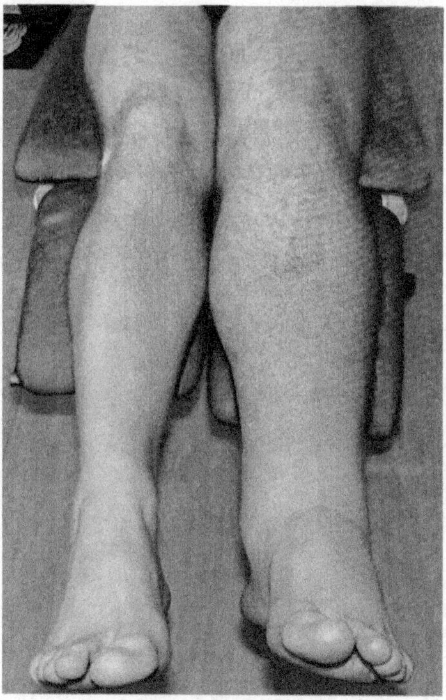

Matt Hazledine – Lymphoedema in left leg, Nov 2011

After hours of research to find help, we told my local Doctor that there was a lymphoedema clinic 10-minutes' drive from my house! He replied *"Oh, I thought that was only for cancer patients."* He referred me to the clinic and a couple of months later, I was under the superb care of an experienced and knowledgeable lymphoedema therapist, Kelly Nickson, who helped to turn my life around.

Kelly listened to my story and provided reassurance that my feelings were normal, post-diagnosis. She gave me helpful information and measured me for bespoke compression garments. Her aim was to reduce the swelling in my left leg from almost 60% bigger in volume than my right leg. To achieve this, she used compression and Complete Decongestive Therapy (CDT) including Multi-Layer Lymphoedema Bandaging (MLLB), and massage using a Compression Pump. At the same time, she was educating me on self-care techniques such as maintaining good skin care, self-massage and living a healthy lifestyle. At its best, my left leg reduced to 35% bigger than my right leg. The problem for me was maintaining that size because my leg always rebounded in between MLLB treatments. I found that even changing to a Class 4S compression stocking, plus a Velcro wrap system didn't have the desired outcome of reducing the size and keeping it that way.

I was soon referred to become a patient of Professor Peter Mortimer, under the NHS at St George's Hospital, London. Under the care of Prof Mortimer and Kelly Nickson, every type of conservative treatment available was tried, which always resulted in only temporary limb reduction. After several tests, including a lymphoscintigraphy – which was very uncomfortable, but fascinating at the same time – it was concluded that surgery would be the only suitable solution for me to reduce the limb size more permanently.

In 2015, I was referred to two surgeons in Essex, England, to perform Lymph Node Transfer surgery. This involved removing cervical lymph nodes from my neck and transferring them to my inguinal nodal area in my groin. After approximately one week in hospital and one month of noticeable limb reduction, my swelling rebounded again. I was so demoralised after such an invasive procedure, which left me with nerve damage in my neck that took years to repair.

Still, not one to give up on me, Professor Mortimer began the investigation into the possibility and suitability of Lymphaticovenular Anastomosis (LVA) and Suction Assisted Protein Lipectomy (SAPL) or Liposuction, as it's often referred to. It transpired, at that time, I wasn't deemed suitable for LVA, so proceeded with SAPL. Dr Kristiana Gordon and her team at St George's Hospital, did an incredible job in securing NHS funding for the surgery and I had liposuction on the lower leg in January 2017 and subsequently on the upper leg in January 2019. I was warned by the surgeon, Katy Milroy, that the pain would be comparable to *"being run over by a bus, twice!".* In truth, I didn't feel a great deal of pain from the liposuction, although my leg was covered in beautifully coloured bruising – green, yellow, and black but no pain!

Now, in 2023, as I write this, my leg is probably down to a size that, although still quite large in the calf, is more much manageable than before my liposuction surgery. I measure my leg in four places on the first day of every month, at the ankle, mid-calf, knee, and mid-thigh and record these measurements on an Excel spreadsheet, so I can monitor size fluctuation much quicker than waiting for my six-month clinic appointment. If my leg is up in size, I use the Velcro wrap system and exercise my legs more, until the volume measurements return to the previous size. It works for me, it might work for you.

I mentioned earlier that I kept my feelings to myself in the early years of lymph-oedema, which in hindsight was not the greatest strategy. I wanted to remain strong and in control to those who knew me; friends, family, work colleagues, but in truth, underneath the brave face I was really struggling to deal with this life-changing disease/condition. I didn't know anyone with lymphoedema, and I just wasn't in the right place to comment or post on the online support groups I'd joined. I buried myself away and only my closest family could really see the effect this was having on my mental health.

It took four years for me to open up about my lymphoedema and, in doing so, I chose to go public with the intention of helping others. My first experience of this was writing a full-page article for the Lymphoedema Support Network (LSN), focusing more on clothing solutions to help others than talking about my personal journey. However, it was a good starting point for me to begin the process of talking about it! I then attended the LSN annual AGM and Patient Day in London and met two other men with lymphoedema, out of approx. 100 attendees, the rest being women, which tells you something, doesn't it? We swapped email addresses and kept in touch, for a while.

I was then persuaded by Professor Mortimer to help raise awareness of lymph-oedema, by telling my story by way of a full-page article in the Good Health section of the Daily Mail. Bizarre, isn't it? I say nothing for years and then choose a national newspaper to share my experiences!

In 2016, I joined the LSN as a Trustee, with the objective of continuing my mission to get the male voice heard, help others, and raise money to support this well-established and well-respected lymphoedema charity. Due to the several surgeries, I'd had, I made the tough decision to stand down in 2018 to focus on my full recovery, family and business.

For almost 12 years, as I write this, I have tried numerous techniques to reduce *and* maintain my swollen leg, in addition to finding clothing and shoe solutions. In 2021, when I was approaching my 10-year anniversary with lymphoedema, (or lymphaversary), I decided to really focus on what had become my passion and purpose. I wanted to create something special to raise awareness around the world, fundraise for several lymphoedema charities and encourage more people (especially men) to talk!

Through my free membership, one-stop-shop patient-based website *www.lymphoedemaunited.com* and my book 'How to Live Better with Lymphoedema – Meet the Experts,' I pass on the countless experiences, solutions and top tips that have worked for me over the years. In addition, both the website and book provide trusted information and guidance from globally recognised lymphoedema experts, with the aim of helping others to live better with lymphoedema.

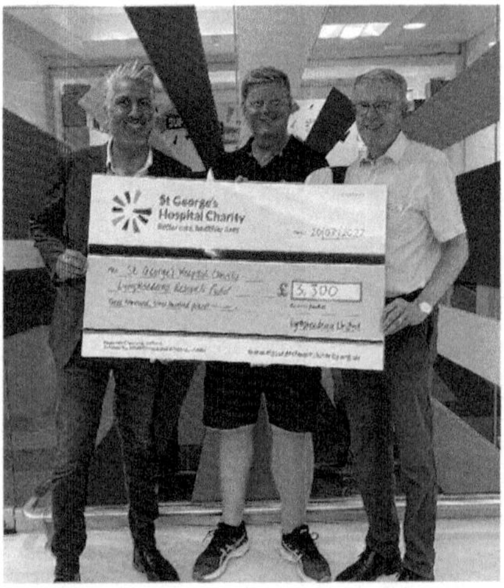

Amerjit Chohan, Matt Hazledine, Prof. Peter Mortimer, 2022

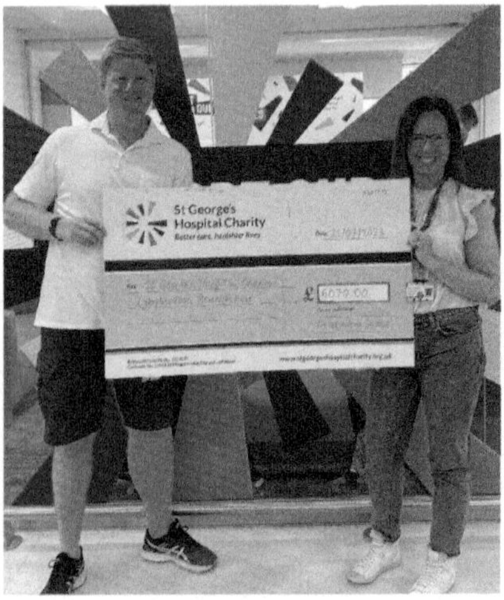

Matt Hazledine & Sarah McCullough, 2023

This has given me the confidence and impetus to create an annual Charity Golf Day, in the UK, to unite golfers with lymphoedema, and/or their loved ones, to play 18 holes with senior management from leading lymphoedema product suppliers and other 'lymphies' (I still don't know if I like that title). In 2022, its first year, we raised £3,300 for the Lymphoedema Research Fund and met new friends for life. In June 2023, 51 people attended our golf day at The Belfry and we raised an incredible £6,070!

Alongside this, I run 'Meet-ups' for locals with lymphoedema in England and I aim to turn this into a national programme. I also post frequently on Facebook, Twitter, Instagram, LinkedIn and have a library of videos and recorded interviews on our YouTube channel. Unite with us @LymphUnited and sign up to our website as a member, free, *www.lymphoedemaunited.com*.

When God gives you lemons, you make lemonade, right?

I hope you are enjoying another one of my projects...this book! Thank you for your support.

TOP TIP!

There are so many people living with lymphoedema who would be there for you, to listen to you, to help you, to understand. Don't bury your head in the sand, like I did. Reach out and talk to someone either online or via a local support group. Always remember, you are NOT alone!

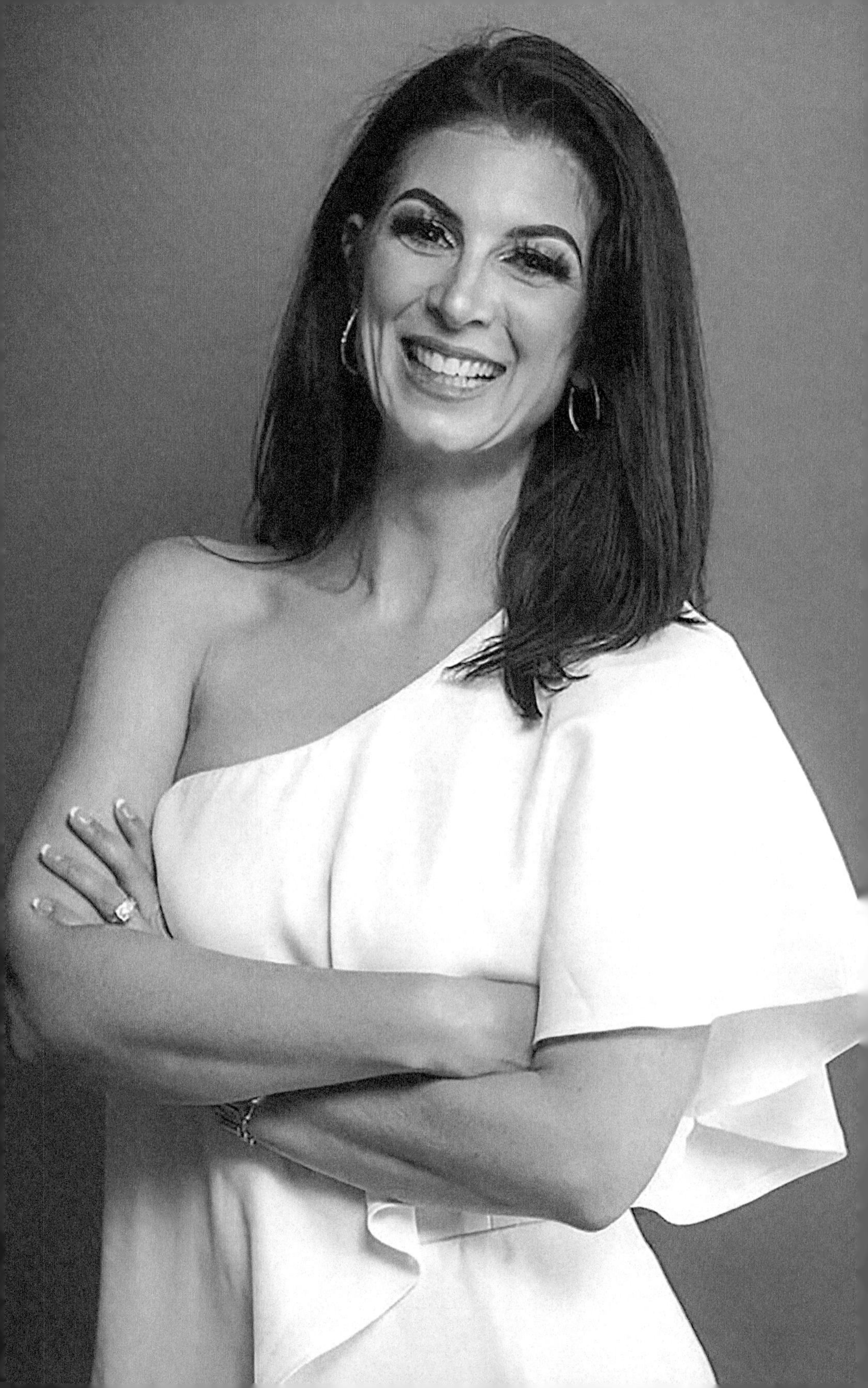

3

AMY RIVERA

> *I persevered in search of a physician who truly understood my struggle and could help me reclaim the life I knew was within me.*

I was born into a world where lymphedema, an incurable condition, cast its heavy shadow upon me, leaving me immensely disfigured. My right leg towered at a staggering 200% larger than my left leg. For the longest time, I carried the weight of isolation and loneliness. Yet, through a lifetime of adversity, I cultivated an activist mindset, tirelessly fighting to improve my quality of life through medicine, nutrition, fitness, and faith. Against insurmountable odds,

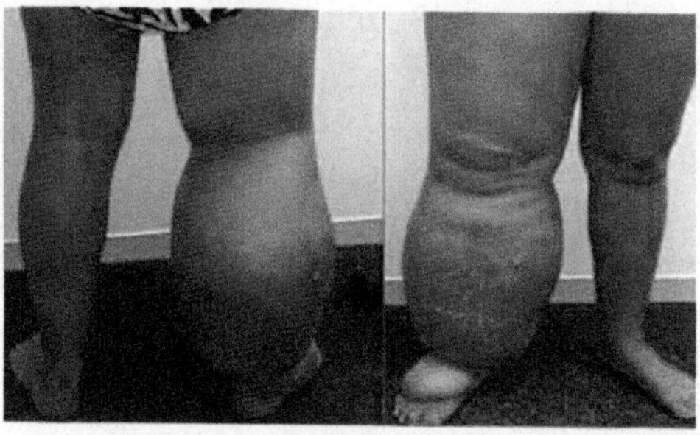

Amy Rivera – Right leg was 200% larger than her left leg

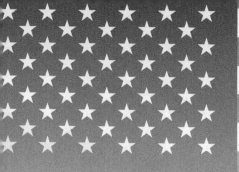

my journey led me to conquer the most severe manifestation of lymphedema, managing it with minimal maintenance.

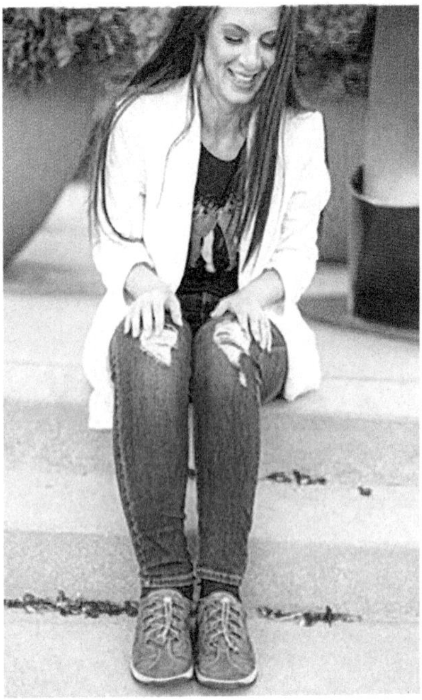
Amy Rivera after surgery in 2018

Though it took me a decade to reach this point, my journey has been one of growth and resilience. From enduring misdiagnoses to failed procedures, I persevered in search of a physician who truly understood my struggle and could help me reclaim the life I knew was within me.

In 2013, I underwent a lymph node transfer, which unfortunately didn't succeed due to the extensive fluid buildup and fibrotic tissue from years of untreated lymphedema. Undeterred, I pursued another surgery called "SAPL" in 2015, only to wake up and discover that a regular liposuction procedure had been performed, leaving me without answers or compression. It was devastating, but I refused to give up. That's when I found Dr. Jay Granzow, and the moment I met him, I knew he was the one. In 2018, the actual SAPL procedure was carried out, and my right leg went from being 200% larger to just 2%! It was an absolute miracle, a testament to the power of perseverance and finding the right doctor who believed in me.

As I gradually opened up about my journey, I started sharing my story with friends, colleagues, and anyone willing to listen. It became a natural instinct to spread awareness and educate others about lymphedema. Before I realized it, my voice was reaching a wider audience, and I found myself sharing my story with the world. It became my purpose, my way of making a difference and raising awareness about this condition.

Throughout more than three decades, I persevered through misdiagnoses and an unyielding pursuit for answers to the persistent swelling that plagued my body. However, within the depths of that struggle, I discovered my purpose and made a solemn vow to dedicate my life to the lymphedema community if I found

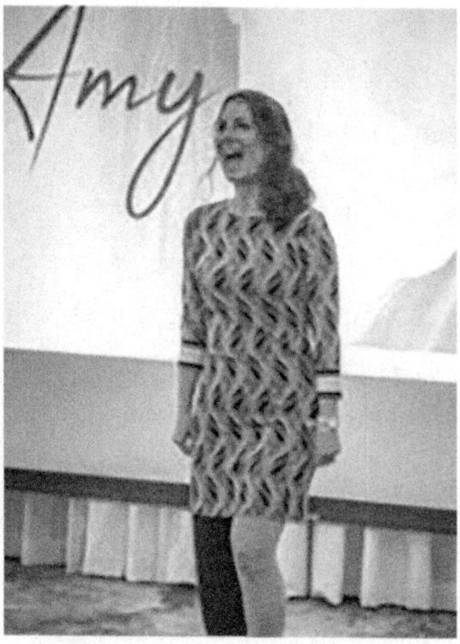

Amy Rivera - Presenting and Inspiring

healing. Determined to make a difference, I left the corporate world behind to answer my calling—to be a voice for those with lymphedema—and to embrace a philanthropic life.

The Lymphedema Treatment Act (LTA) is a crucial piece of legislation aimed at improving access to comprehensive lymphedema treatment for all individuals in the United States. The LTA advocates for insurance coverage of compression. By lobbying for the LTA in Washington DC, we sought to raise awareness about the importance of proper treatment and support for individuals living with lymphedema. After 12 years of relentless efforts, I am overjoyed to announce that the LTA has been passed and will go into effect starting January 2024. This landmark achievement will bring hope and relief to countless individuals across the country, ensuring they have the resources and support they need to manage their lymphedema effectively.

Today, as the founder of the Ninjas Fighting Lymphedema Foundation, I stand at the helm of a powerful movement that empowers individuals battling lymphedema to embrace their inherent strength and resilience. Through unwavering support, comprehensive education, and tireless advocacy, we strive to make a profound and positive impact in their lives while raising widespread awareness about this often-misunderstood condition.

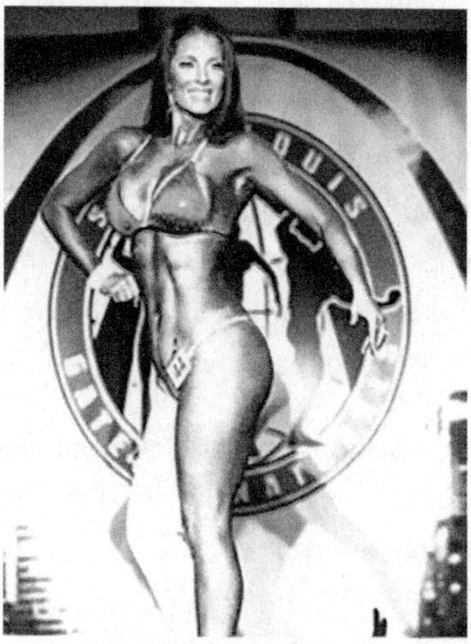

Amy Rivera - Bodybuilder

Despite lymphedema taking away my childhood, it has bestowed upon me invaluable gifts in adulthood. Those who know me are aware of my passion for sports, and one of my childhood aspirations was to compete in a bodybuilding competition.

Not only did I want to test my mental fortitude, but I also cherished the time spent in the gym. In 2021, I proudly stepped onto the stage and achieved the remarkable feat of securing 3rd and 4th place in the competition.

In alignment with my unwavering commitment, I established Rivera Hybrid Solutions—a pioneering company exclusively focused on developing groundbreaking solutions for lymphedema management. Our flagship product, the Fast'n Go Hybrid Compression Bandages, represents a significant breakthrough. These single-layer, multi-component hybrid bandages are meticulously designed for self-bandaging, delivering unparalleled comfort and efficacy. By placing control back into the hands of individuals, we empower them to take charge of their lymphedema care journey.

Beyond my entrepreneurial pursuits, I am the driving force behind the Lymphedema Blueprint Course—a comprehensive program that guides individuals through every facet of their lymphedema journey. From gaining a profound understanding of the condition to effectively managing symptoms and maintaining overall wellness, this transformative course equips participants with invaluable knowledge and practical tools for living a fulfilling life.

As the author of the inspiring memoir "Drop The Skirt: How My Disability Became My Superpower," I wholeheartedly share my personal story of resilience and self-acceptance. The front cover of my book serves as a symbol of liberation, representing the profound shift in my mindset—from concealing my lymphedema to fearlessly raising awareness about it. I had to release the shackles of judgment imposed by others and focus on how I perceived myself, ultimately embracing my uniqueness and reclaiming my power.

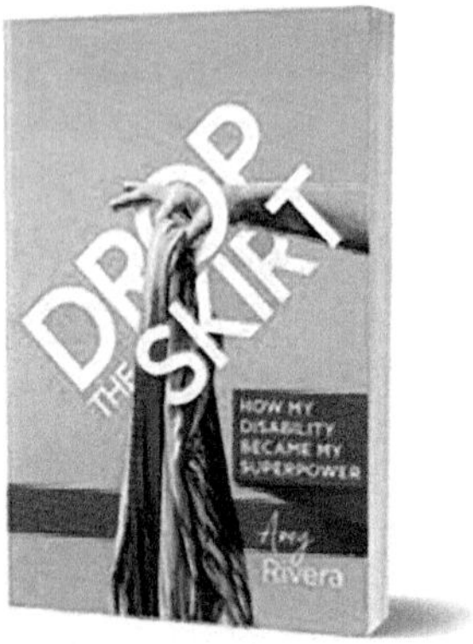

Amy Rivera - Drop the Skirt

However, my journey extends far beyond my personal experiences. It encompasses my daughter, who battles lymphedema and lipedema. Through unwavering advocacy and dedication, I have shed light on these conditions within my own family, fostering awareness that transcends generations. Jade courageously shares her personal journey in this book.

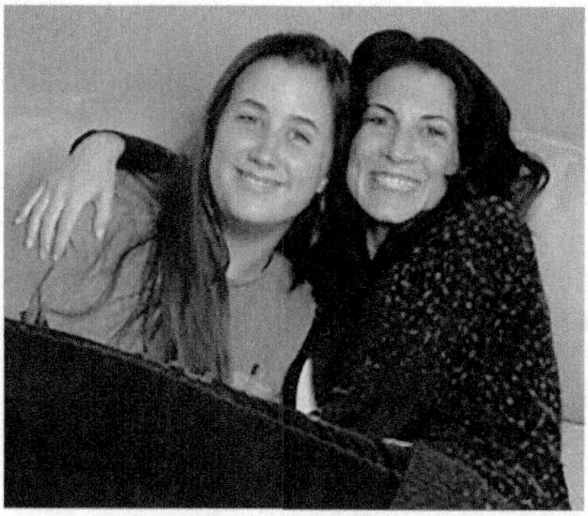
Amy Rivera - with daughter Jade

Within this anthology, we unite not only to raise awareness within our immediate community but also to leave an enduring legacy of hope for future generations. We deeply understand the incredible power of storytelling—to inspire, educate, and uplift others. Through the collective sharing of our stories, we shatter barriers, debunk misconceptions, and demonstrate to others that they are never alone on their journey.

I want to express my heartfelt gratitude to everyone who has bravely shared their own stories. Your courage ignites a beacon.

TOP TIP!

Prioritize self-care and find what works best for you. This may include implementing a consistent lymphedema management routine, staying active, maintaining a healthy lifestyle, seeking support from others, and advocating for your own needs. Remember, you are the expert of your own body and it's important to listen to it and take care of yourself.

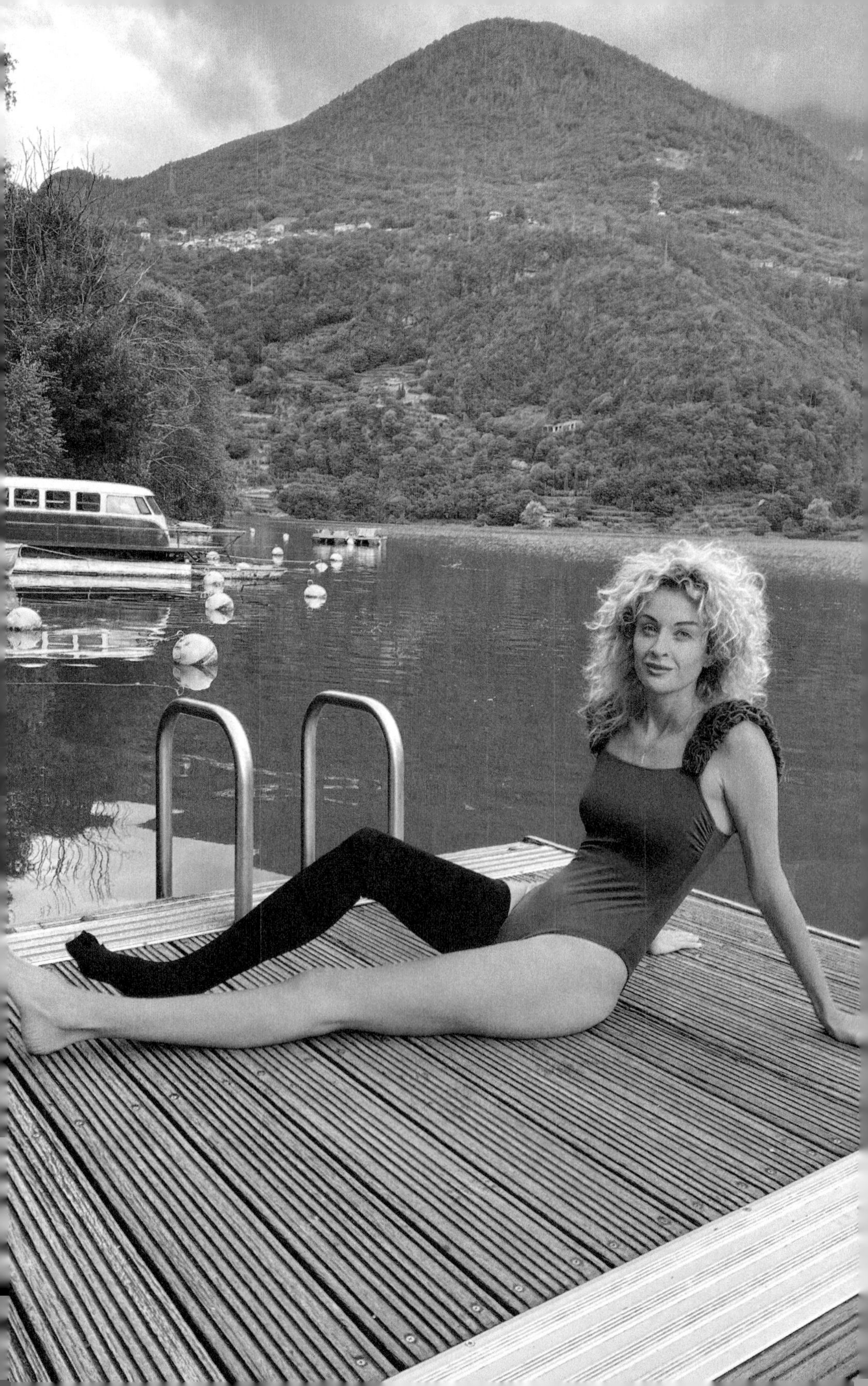

4

ANNA MAISETTI

> ***I tried to hide my leg in every way to avoid questions, even going so far as to avoid going out.***

My name is Anna Maisetti, I'm 35 and I'm Italian. At the age of 22, during a waxing session, the beautician pointed out to me a small swelling on the skin, similar to a mole which, in a short time, changed color and shape; first pink, then black, and finally gray. At the time I was not attentive to prevention: I subjected myself to the sun's rays without protection and often resorted to lamps. I randomly looked for a dermatologist for an aesthetic consultation, who did not recognize the seriousness of the situation and advised me to have it removed without urgency, with the times of the Health System. Thus 12 months have passed and, when the histological examination was done, the reality turned out to be much more serious.

It was a malignant tumor of the skin and, after various examinations and investigations, it was discovered that it had already reached the lymph nodes in the

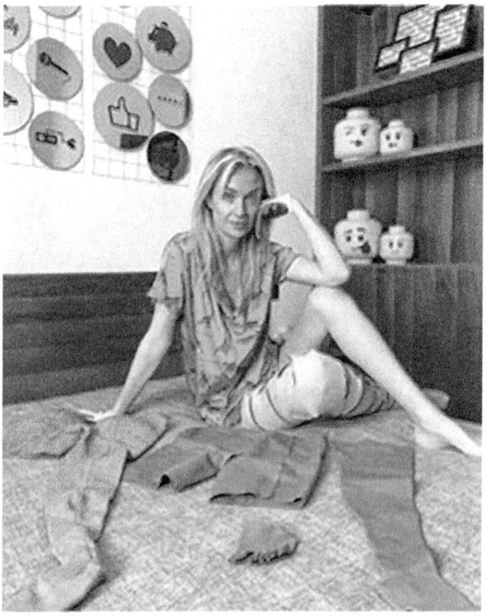

right groin which, after various tests, were removed. The consequence was to develop a chronic, disabling, and evolutionary pathology, which is called lymphedema. It was a real shock and a radical life change. All in no time.

For eight years I went through all of this in hiding because I was ashamed of my new body.

I was a girl who loved miniskirts and high heels and I found myself having to constantly wear unsightly and rigid medical stockings, even in the summer, and to endure heavy bandages, which do not allow the wearing of common shoes. I tried to hide my leg in every way to avoid questions, even going so far as to avoid going out.

Furthermore, I did not know anyone in the same condition and, even in the therapeutic process and in the recognition of the disability, I encountered many obstacles due to the lack of awareness of this problem. For example, getting a custom-made stocking with the characteristics indicated by the doctor was an odyssey and an incredible waste of time and money, or, in some situations, this pathology was even confused and belittled. Luckily, in all of this, I have always had an understanding family and friends by my side, employers who have been close to me along this journey, also made up of countless absences, and professionals I met along the way, who have been real "angels".

In a moment of great discouragement, I thought it wasn't possible that only I was suffering from it, and I was facing such a difficult path, I understood that Instagram with search via # could be the best way to connect with other people. Furthermore, I felt the need to reach out to anyone who was at the beginning of this "adventure" or who hadn't yet found a diagnosis, to make many phases that I had already faced and overcome less painful and easier, and to disseminate information, creating a network that it didn't exist. I named my page "stile_compresso"

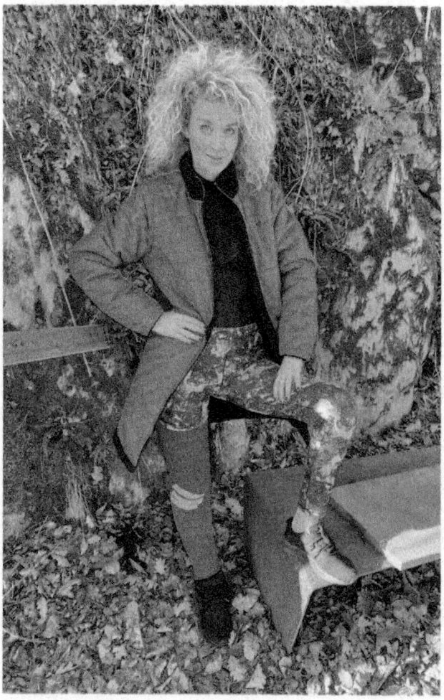

Stile(Style): for sharing lifestyle and information that revolves inexorably around the leg, but also to convey a message related to inclusive fashion, not only as practical and necessary advice to deal with the needs of an asymmetrical and delicate body but to spread an idea of uniqueness, especially on Instagram, where most profiles flaunt a perfection that doesn't exist. The goal is also to break down all those stereotypes about bodies that don't take into account the precious characteristics that differentiate each of us.

(Compresso) Compress: to recall the need to always wear socks, bandages, and braces that I prefer colored and decorated as a symbol of "never giving up" and always reacting to life's difficulties.

To date, the community has more than 22,000 people, who follow the shares of various types with interest. My experience and my knowledge have been enriched, allowing me to become an increasingly expert patient thanks to the meetings and collaborations with some of the most important international professors and scholars. I had the honor of telling my story to the Ministry of Health, representing patients at the opening of an important conference held in Dubai, and of working with some professors on a project with Standford University.

I spoke to young people in universities and took part in events dedicated to personal growth and inclusion; moreover, I wrote the book "Lymphedema after Cancer", available only on Amazon, which has been translated into Italian, English, and German; I created a video, involving a hundred patients and professionals from all over the world to celebrate International Lymphoedema Day, which takes place on March 06 of each year; I collaborate with the Airc association as an ambassador, to support research; I took part in the Body Positive Cat Walk in Milan and opened the Defilet della Rinascita event on the Bassano bridge, parading hand in hand with 40 other women operated on for cancer. Finally, I was chosen for an international fashion campaign by photographer Mihaela Noroc and I was given the opportunity to design t-shirts for a well-known brand, which were sold for charity.

Hundreds of patients, thanks to sharing, have found information, deepening their path and even finding a diagnosis, and have had the courage to expose themselves and show themselves as they are. These experiences, together with many others, have allowed me to create important and precious friendships all over the world and also to have extra work opportunities for my beloved job, which allow me to express my creativity and my style in different forms. If I had continued to hide, this never would have happened.

The cause that is closest to my heart concerns children. In Italy, there is a small but important Association, based in Piemonte, called Lymphido, founded by parents of young patients, sponsored by ITALF. Every year it organizes summer camps for children and families struggling with pediatric lymphedema, allowing them to experience three days of fun, friendship and, above all, providing help and important teachings.

I'm proud of the impact we've made, providing support, awareness, and unity to hundreds of patients. Together, we've created a network that didn't exist before, empowering individuals to embrace their uniqueness. Additionally, I continue to advocate for research and work with various organizations to make a difference.

TOP TIP!

Embrace color, style, and confidence in your lymphedema journey. Dare to dress your leg or arm with vibrant fashion, conveying a message of resilience and personal expression. Don't fear to always dare!

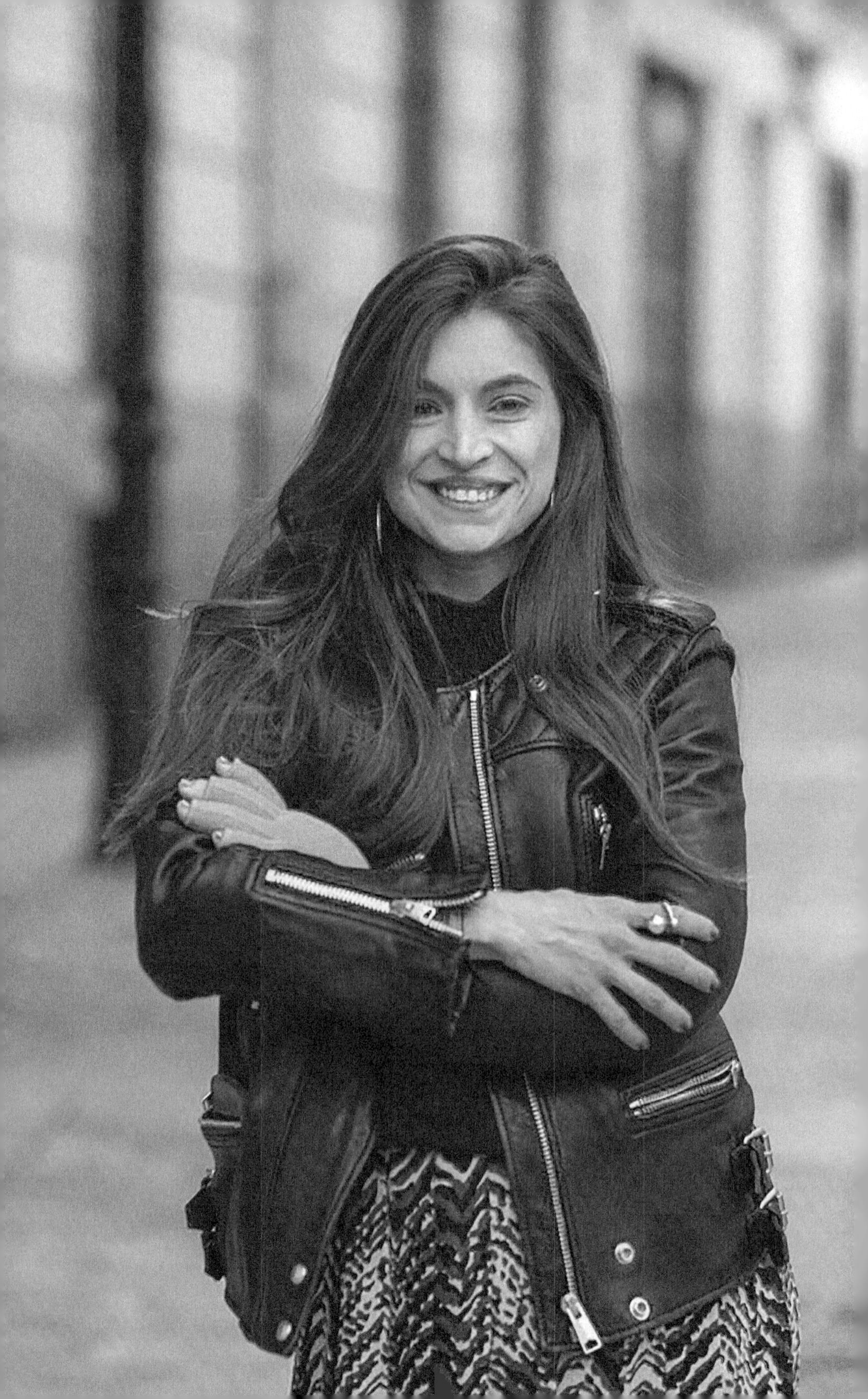

5

NICOLE FACCIO

> ***I wanted to ignore my reality and demonstrate to everyone that I was as 'normal' as them.***

In the summer of 2018, 6 months after I had moved to London, I had to commute for almost 3 hours daily to work for a client. The daily travel consisted of a bus, a tube, another tube, a train and a shuttle in order to get to the client's office. I can hear the panic gasp from any Lymphedema patient after that sentence. Yes, it was a lot.

I was not happy with this, as I had sworn after 5 years of living in New York and putting my body through a lot of hecticness that deteriorated my health, sometimes even having to travel out of state for work, that I was not going to submit myself to such stress and strain EVER AGAIN! I was adamant that I was going to prioritize my health and that anything that put me in a position where I had to neglect my Lymphedema maintenance, would have to come to an end immediately. I was in the mindset that Lymphedema care was my first priority because that had returned my ability to enjoy a good quality of life after a very dark time, and if that meant for me to ask for accommodations at work, I would.

Prior to this, I feared requesting such things because I was worried it would come off as "weak" or "lazy", or that showing my vulnerability could have consequences on my career. I was too proud to accept that I might need some type of workplace accommodation, even when early on in my career I started to notice that my Lymphedema was progressing fast and with a vengeance.

Believe me, the word Lymphedema wouldn't come out of my mouth at work. I was working at a top consulting firm, and I was the only woman out of 6 hired from my university. I had a job offer 6 months before graduating which is an incredible achievement. Failing was not an option. Back then I would think of any type of arrangement as a "special treatment", and anything special like this was frowned upon. I was not equipped in setting boundaries because there was no such thing back then, although I no longer blame myself for this mentality because it is truly corporate America's fault for the unattainable standard of productivity and quite honestly ridiculous definition of success. But here I was, subscribed to the system and living in one of the most complicated and workaholic cities in the world. And I wanted to compete and be competitive just like everyone else around me. I wanted to ignore my reality and demonstrate to everyone that I was as "normal" as them, that I didn't have challenges and that my swollen arm was just something I was born with, not something that affected me in any other way. Or maybe, I was trying to prove that to myself. In fact, for 3 years I never told anyone at work about Lymphedema. Jokes on me honestly because it is not like I can really hide my Lymphedema from me or from anyone else.

This deserves a bit of context, in case you don't know me. My name is Nicole Faccio, and I was born with a rare genetic disorder called the WILD syndrome - which I thought was Milroy's Disease until 2 years ago. WILD syndrome causes lymphatic abnormalities in your whole lymphatic system that results in a chronic accumulation of fluid that therefore results in the Lymphedema. The definition criteria of the clinical syndrome is the presence of **W**arts, **I**mmunodeficiency, **L**ymphoedema and anogenital **D**ysplasia. Because of this I have a collapsed left lung, Lymphedema in my left arm, both my legs, abdomen and genitals, a little bit in my face, as well as protein losing enteropathy in my digestive system which probably means I have a central lymphatics issue too. I've had Lymphedema since the moment of birth, so the reality is that I don't know a life without it. Of course, not to the extent of what I live with now, but chronic swelling has always been part of my body and my day-to-day. During my childhood and my adolescence my Lymphedema was fairly stable, probably because of the incredible maintenance routine my parents had incorporated into my life, and it wasn't until my early adulthood, around my early 20s, that I started experiencing the exhaustion, heaviness and physical limitations of the condition. To be honest, no one had really told us that the Lymphedema could progress if left untreated, and I took a lot of liberties in my younger years that I now understand were quite harmful to my health. Just as an example, I probably didn't wear a compression garment for maybe 4 or 5 years on my arm. I also did not consistently start wearing compression on my legs until I was 22 years old. I developed some type of antagonism against the care of Lymphedema because I used a pneumatic machine for 17 years which ended up being the cause of my pleural effusion that collapsed my lung, and genital lymphedema.

I often thought I could give Lymphedema a little bit of care and that'll be enough to continue on until I decided I'll give it a little more extra care. Of course, I was wrong, and I am grateful I live to tell the tale.

I neglected the condition and deprioritised it completely. I wanted to live and see the world, and I did. Of course, this had its consequences as Lymphedema will claim its space in your body and so it did in mine. Therefore, in 2016, I found myself putting a pause in the life and career I had built in NYC to go to Germany for a 2-month treatment and had surgery for my genital edema. This period of my life turned it all around, reason I call it my *Lymphie Saturn Return*. It taught me everything I know and gave me back my life, something I'll be completely indebted to everyone that participated in that part of my journey.

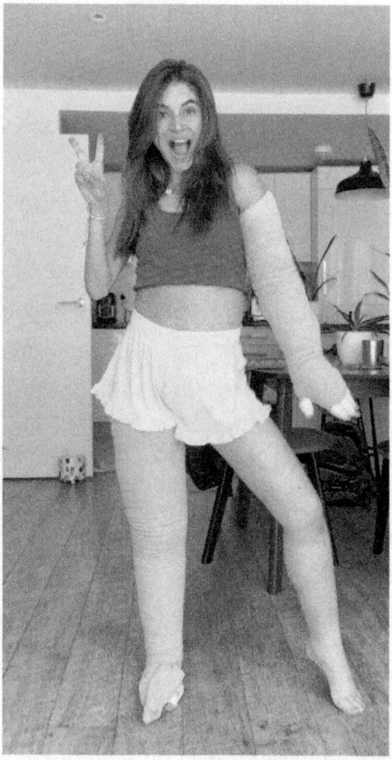

Nicole Faccio – That's a wrap!

So, now back in 2018, the stability and the maintenance protocol I fought so hard to incorporate into my life had become super sacred to me. This change in lifestyle also meant that I was strict about the way I ate. I was not going to let anyone or anything interfere with that. I had stared in the eyes of my biggest fear of getting to the end of my functional life and realized I had been given another chance in life, and I was not going to throw that away. But here came my job, putting me in a tough position again. This time around it was up to me to establish those boundaries. I asked for the "accommodations" this time, but it still required for me to do that same level of travel at least 3 times a week, and with time it proved to be more and more challenging. I was very paranoid that all my progress during the last 2 years was going to be lost. I was about to ask to be taken out of the role but luckily a very magical thing happened.

A random day towards the end of summer, I was eating in the cafeteria at the dreaded client's office, and I saw this man from a distance with a black sleeve on his arm. I swear I probably did like a triple take to make sure I was seeing properly. And I was! I know the compression products very well so I could recognise the brand and knit quality from afar, so I knew I had probably spotted another Lymphie in the building. I don't know if you have ever been in this position, but this is like finding a rare Pokémon moment. I probably looked like a stalker walking slyly around the cafeteria. People must have thought I was being rude because I was explicitly staring. But I was just in shock and trying to figure out either my entry or next steps.

I was on my way out to the toilet, so I decided to continue my way as he was sitting on the table having lunch with other people and I didn't want to interrupt. I orchestrated in my head what my opening line was going to be: "Hey, I think we have a matching fashion sense"... nailed it!

I quickly went to the toilet and came back in a rush to approach him and see if he was free (no, I didn't wash my hands, this was pre-covid and what arm Lymphies do, pfttt). To my misfortune he was still with his co-workers. I was desperate to not miss him and to talk to him but did that anxious thing of walking around "discreetly" but at an accelerated pace. Came back 5 min later – still busy. UGH!

Then, a co-worker of mine saw me and started discussing some work matters with me, which I couldn't tell you what it was about because I paid no attention since my mind was on a Lymphie mission. The chit chat lasted for a while, so when I was able to disengage and check again on the Lymphie, he was gone.

GUTTED! I swear I did a couple of laps around the several floors and meeting rooms and didn't find him. I was so annoyed, but duty called, and I went back to work with the hopes that I would see him again eventually.

A couple of months later, still commuting and pushing to get out of the role, although everyone wanted me to stay, I found myself late for a meeting, as per usual, and running up the stairs, when I saw my mystery Lymphie coming down. With the same rush and urgency, I was running up I stopped, turned around and grabbed him and said, "Oh hey, what happened to your arm?"

Mystery Lymphie looked at me with a deer in headlights face and then I realized what I had just asked. That same question I hated to be asked all these years but often got. Oops!

Mystery Lymphie: "That's a private matter, please respect it"

Nicole: No! I'm sorry I have it too! Pointing to my arm with a black garment too.

Mystery Lymphie looked even more perplexed than before

Mystery Lymphie: "Do you have Lymphoedema?" (British spelling of course)

Nicole: "Yes!"

Mystery Lymphie: "I have it in my legs too"

Nicole: "Me too!"

The conversation continued, but I'd be lying if I told you exactly how it went. I just remember it was beautiful, chaotic, and dramatic. I will always remember it fondly. We then exchanged emails so we could continue this conversation at another time. I'll maintain the name of Mystery Lymphie anonymously, but I have a lot to thank him for.

First, he gave me the name of the doctors at St Georges, the main Lymphedema clinic in the UK and in London. Funnily enough, the place that originated the research and wrote the paper on WILD syndrome.

Second, that moment made me realize I was meant to be on that client site, regardless of the effort of the commute. Coincidences like that are not coincidences, they are signs. Or so I like to think.

Third, this was the second time in my life I randomly met a Lymphie, and in similar ways those experiences had a profound impact on the trajectory of my life. It made me feel that every previous step I had taken was perfectly aligned for me to be there in that moment, to be here in London, for a reason. Mystery Lymphie and I had so many things in common, we were around the same age with the same diagnosis and experienced similar challenges throughout our lives. It's now hard to believe that I thought I was on my own all this time. It's remarkable to realize now that I wasn't the only one experiencing this all along.

From that moment on I started brainstorming and cooking what a year later became an Instagram takeover that never stopped, in addition to the idea of Normal Adjustments, my podcast. Moments like this have made me realize I was luckier than what I thought, because the universe was conspiring for me, not against me like I once thought.

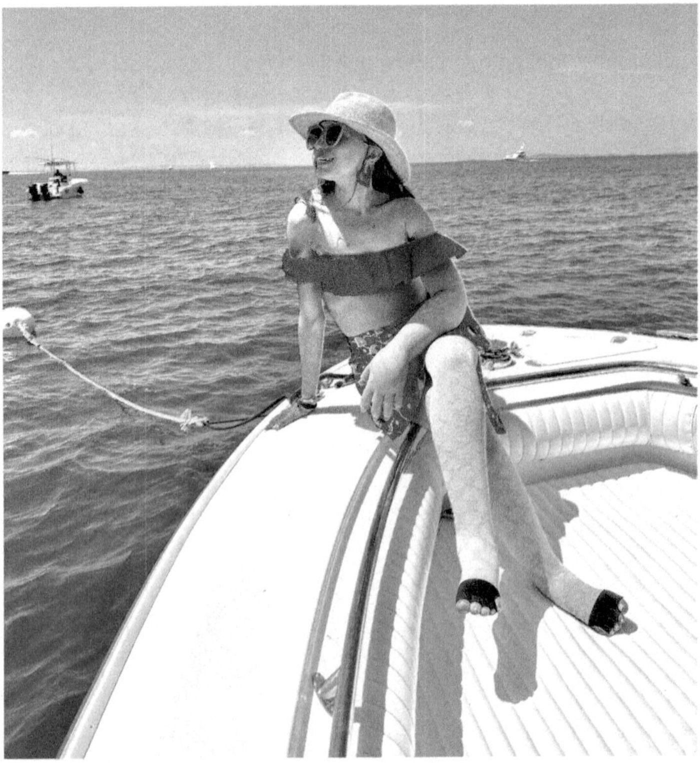

Nicole Faccio - Just making 'Normal Adjustments.'

I guess that life works in mysterious ways, and if you find yourself reading this you might feel distraught, frustrated, and sad because lymphedema happened to you. I understand that I honestly do because I did think that too. I hated everything about it. Then life gave me the gift of understanding perception and gave me hints that made me realize that Lymphedema was not something negative that just happened to me. It was the *adjustment* that was assigned to me, just like many other adjustments are assigned to everyone in the world. Our realities vary so much and what we have as humans is the ability to share and empathize over each of our own adjustments. There is no need to feel shame for it because we all have them. The adjustments make us, us. They make us unique and beautiful.

It is crazy to think that something I neglected about myself for so long, I've now developed such a gratitude towards. Lymphedema has given me a life purpose, a sense of belonging and a purpose of living, and I'm grateful for my annoying, stubborn adjustment.

The road to acceptance is not easy nor short, but I assure you that when you go through that door, it shuts right behind you to never look back. With adjustments and all.

TOP TIP!

Wear your compression!

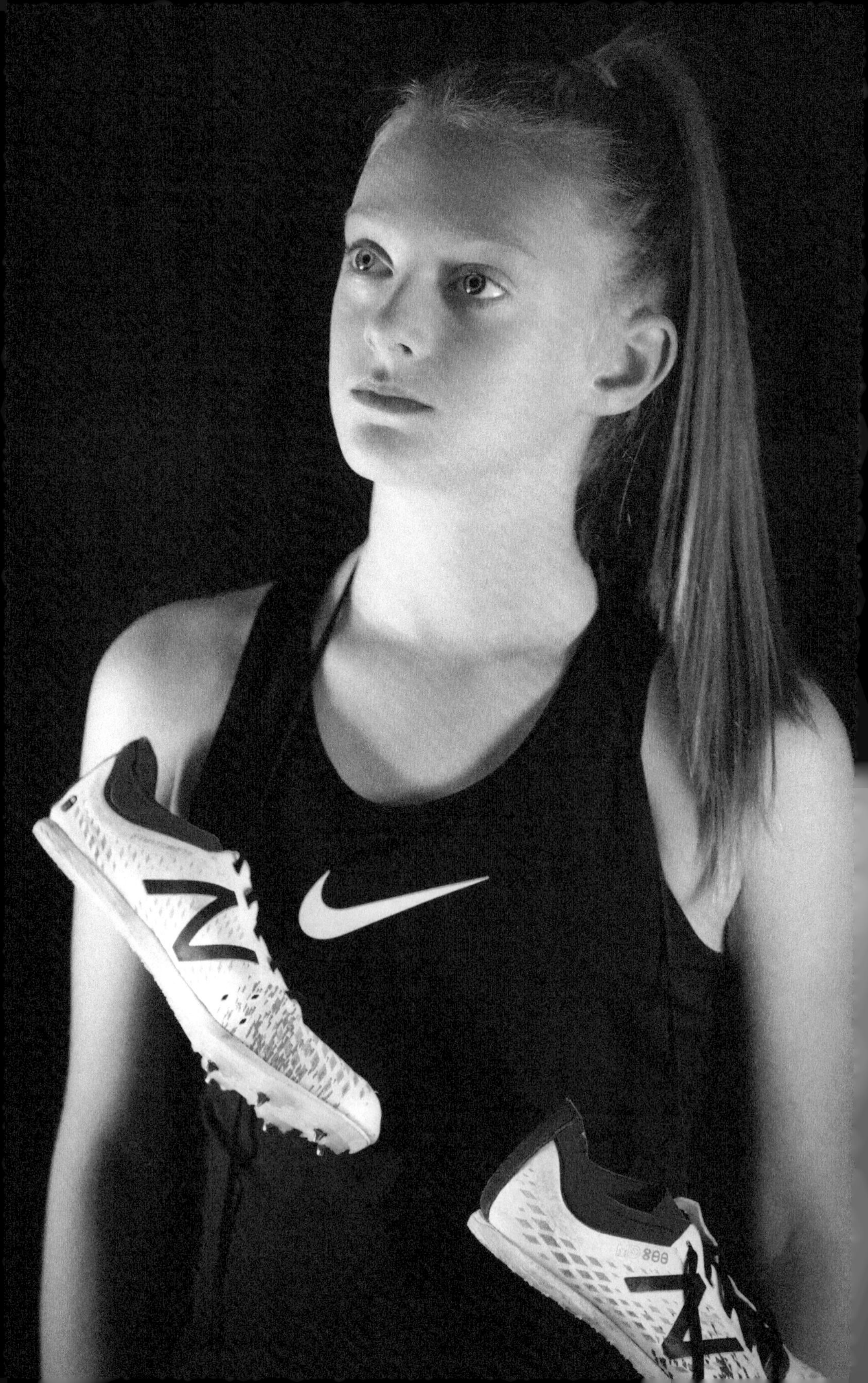

6

LIV LAVANDER

> *Lymphoedema – Never heard of it!*

I am 15 years old as I write this, and I share my story with the aim of helping others to not feel alone.

Just after my 13th Birthday in October 2020 and during the Covid-19 lockdown, I noticed a strange swelling in my lower abdomen which was slightly towards the left.

I remember calling for my Mum to take a look. She asked the usual questions... Does it hurt? Have you banged it on anything? Etc. However, it didn't hurt at all. I couldn't remember injuring it on anything, but it is quite possible as I took part in various sports from hockey, netball, cross country running to athletics, dance, horse-riding, and horse vaulting. Basically, you name the sport, I've done it.

The next day, my Mum took another look and decided to call the Doctor. As it was during lockdown and there were many restrictions, she had to request a call back from them. As a result of the telephone call with them, they decided I needed to go to the Doctor's surgery for them to take a look.

We saw a senior partner at the practice, who asked me to provide a urine sample there and then. Fortunately, that was clear of any infection. He then examined my tummy and got me to cough. He said he was going to ask a colleague to also take a look, as he was a little baffled. After her examination, she was also baffled. Initially they mentioned it could be a hernia. They discussed with mum that they thought it was best to get it checked out at our local hospital, Birmingham Children's Hospital, and sent us home. As it was uncertain times during lockdown, he was unsure what the timescale or situation was with regards to appointments.

He called mum the next morning and said to go straight to A&E as they were expecting me. After arriving there, we first saw a triage nurse who asked lots of questions and told me I couldn't eat or drink anything. She also put some numbing gel on my hand, took my weight and sent us back into the waiting area.

When we finally went through to see the doctor, I remember a nurse wanted to take some blood!!!!! What an experience that was! She tried a million places to get it from me and I just remember having a complete meltdown and wanting to go home there and then. *'My lump wasn't hurting me, so why were they hurting me?',* was my thought at that time.

A Doctor came to see me and examined the lump. She also looked very puzzled and also sent for a 'friend' to come and take a look. They both agreed that I needed an ultrasound, and so off I went to a different part of the hospital. I had the scan and waited for a member of the surgical team to view them. In total I was there for about 11 hours and was literally starving as I still couldn't eat. I remember my Dad dropping off some things for us but he wasn't allowed in, as covid rules were very strict then.

The doctor that sent me for the scan was in theatre, so we had to wait for him to come out and look at the scans. Another doctor eventually came to speak to us and said there wasn't a hernia, but they were still unsure what it was as there was swelling showing up on the scan. They kept asking if I'd injured it on anything, for example, playing sport. The answer was still no!

The Doctor explained that, sometimes, during puberty (but mainly in boys) you can have swelling that will just go in time. I could tell Mum wasn't too happy with this explanation!

She said I could go home and they would book another appointment, via telephone, with a member of the surgical team in three weeks, but obviously if things change I had to go straight back to A&E.

The appointment came and Mum had the telephone call with the Doctor, and once again it was decided that he needed to examine me.

A face-to-face appointment was booked with the Doctor around a week later. Again, he wasn't sure what this lump was and gave us no concrete answers. He looked at the scans again and said it just showed oedema. He said it wasn't anything nasty such as cancer, which was a huge relief, but he still wasn't sure. He sent us away and booked another appointment for us about 6 weeks later to see if there was any change.

At the next appointment, I saw a different doctor with a few student doctors, who again looked at the scans and notes and examined me and said I was a bit of a mystery to them. She decided that instead of calling me back every few months, they would sign me off for a year and if anything changed, I should go straight back! Again, Mum didn't seem too impressed with this.

About three weeks later, I went on a very long bike ride with my Mum, Dad and some friends around Birmingham. Literally, the following day the swelling had gone into the top of my left thigh. I was home-schooling with my Nan looking after me, as Mum was at work. I think Nan must have called Mum to tell her and she came home immediately and took me straight to A&E. Luckily, we didn't have to go through the long process as before, as mum explained that I was under the surgical team, so they just called for one of the team to come down and see me.

I saw yet another doctor, who said I needed a biopsy and MRI scan, but he would talk to the doctor in charge of my case the following day to see what he thought first.

My MRI was booked in for 3 weeks later, and that was on the emergency list! They also booked a biopsy but had to wait for scan first. Luckily, I didn't have to have the biopsy.

After another few weeks, I went back to see the doctor for the scan results. He said he could cut into my leg, but it wouldn't necessarily give him any more answers. He said it could be a lymphatic malformation that was present from birth, and I'd not known about it until now... Mum was having none of that!

He said he'd refer us to the Interventional Radiologist to see if they could help further and the Multi-Disciplinary Team would also be involved.

In between this time, I was sent for a lymphoscintigram to look at the lymph flow in both legs from the toes up. That was the most painful thing... those injections between my toes – brutal!

Mum got in touch with a private Interventional Radiologist, who was a friend of a friend to see if he could help. He also worked part time at the Children's Hospital and said next time he was there he would take our case to the MDT and follow it through for me. He did just that and ended up helping us no end. He scanned me again and said the MRI showed possible blockage in my groin, which could be a blood clot. He then did another ultrasound and suggested a venogram to be 100% sure. My first general anaesthetic – not pleasant coming round! I'd gone from a healthy, sporty fit child who had never had many illnesses/problems to having all this done! Ian, our Interventional Radiographer, had also spoken to a colleague in London who suggested the next step should be a referral to see a Lymphoedema Specialist in either Derby or London. We decided that Derby would be easier to get to, so we booked an appointment to see Professor Vaughan Keeley.

During the appointment, I was measured up for school tights – with compression in the left leg only, but I hated wearing these with a passion.

After Professor Keeley looked at the scans from Birmingham Hospital, he sent me for another ultrasound at the Royal Derby Hospital, as he had a colleague there who really knew what and where to look. He spoke to us throughout the scan and showed us exactly where and what the problem was. The lymph nodes in my left groin looked completely non-existent and blurry compared to the crisp crescent shaped ones on the right. At long last, we felt like we were getting somewhere as I had a diagnosis of lymphoedema.

We had another appointment to see Professor Keeley, who explained that my type of Lymphoedema could be potentially operated on, but only privately at

Oxford Lymphoedema Practice, and with no guarantee of success, although I could apply for funding. I also had to have a test first to see if I could actually have the operation which was also quite expensive.

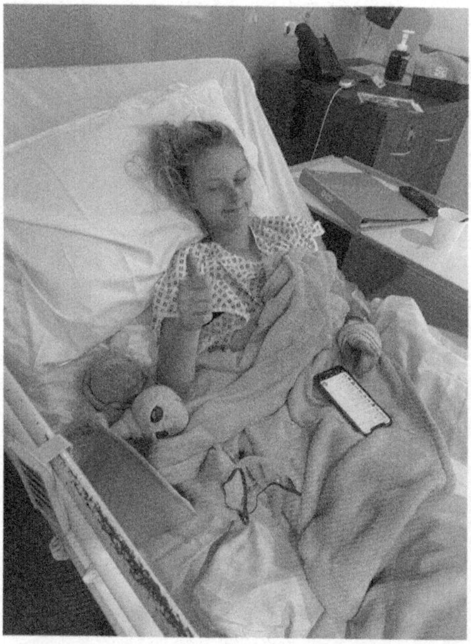

Liv Lavander – LVA Surgery June 2022

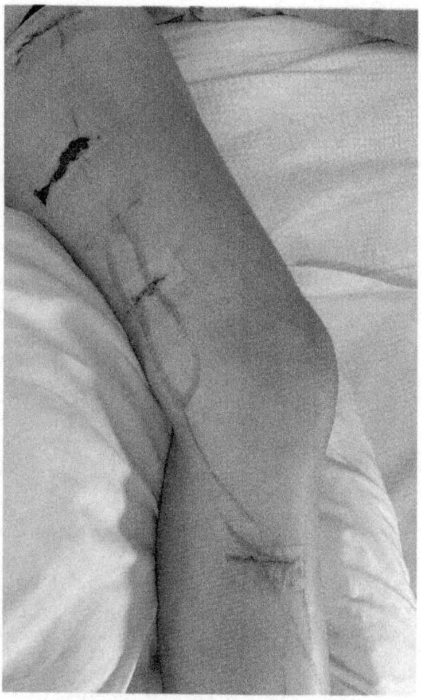

Liv Lavander – LVA Surgery June 2022

After I had that test, I had the operation on 28th June 2022. Professor Furniss performed the Lymphaticovenular Anastomosis (LVA) surgery. He connected the lymph vessels to the veins to try and bypass the blockage and keep the lymph moving. I have four biggish scars on the inside of my leg but I'm proud of them. It shows that something is actually wrong with my leg, rather than people thinking I've just got a fat leg.

6-months after surgery, my leg had reduced by 6%, which is not a massive reduction, but it's no bigger which is the main thing. My next appointment with Professor Furniss is in June 2023 and I'll also have one at the Derby Hospital then too.

Before the operation, I would be embarrassed to show my leg and have photos taken. I hated wearing compression for sport, as I didn't want to look different from my friends who just wore normal PE kit. I used to wear tracksuit bottoms, even in hot weather, rather than my skort (Skirt/Short). I also had to stop hurdles in athletics as I didn't know if that was affecting the lymphoedema in my leg.

To try and get back to my normal life, I have recently joined a ladies hockey Team which I absolutely love. We train on Wednesdays and have fixtures every Saturday. I also compete with my pony in competitions all over the country. I am also taking PE as one of my GCSE exams and my chosen sports are Dance, Hockey and Netball.

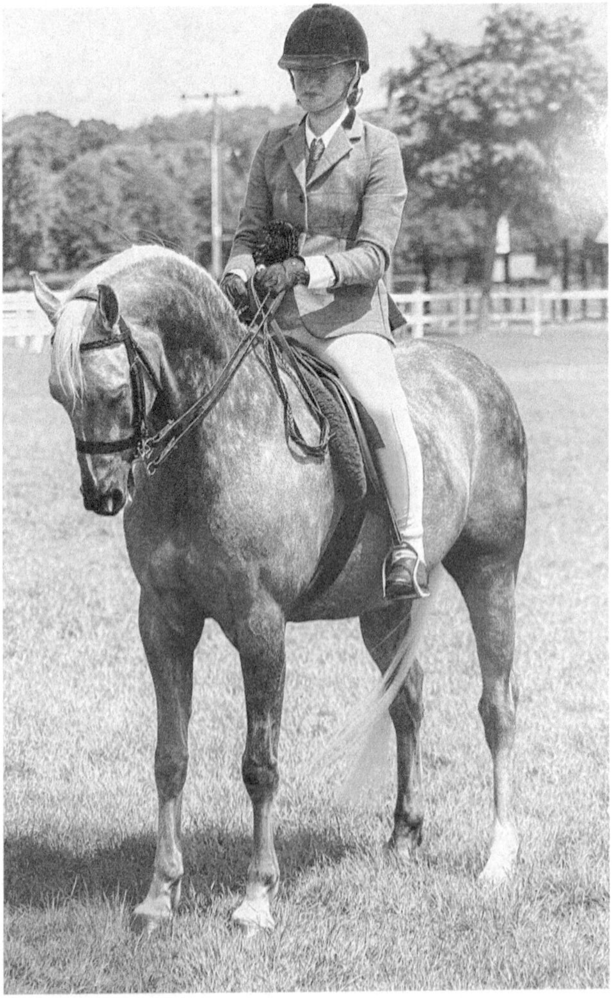

Liv Lavander - Competing in competitions with her Pony, Henry

So, my top tip would be to never give up asking for answers. My Mum pushed and pestered weekly to get my diagnosis. The time it took was ridiculous. We could see my leg growing in front of our eyes and no one was telling us what it was, what to do, or taking on my case. We were pushed from one department to the next until we were referred to see Professor Keeley, where we got a diagnosis, treatment and advice. This has enabled me to get on with my life again and do the sports I love, like most teenagers.

TOP TIP!

Never give up asking for answers!
If surgery is right for you, have it done.

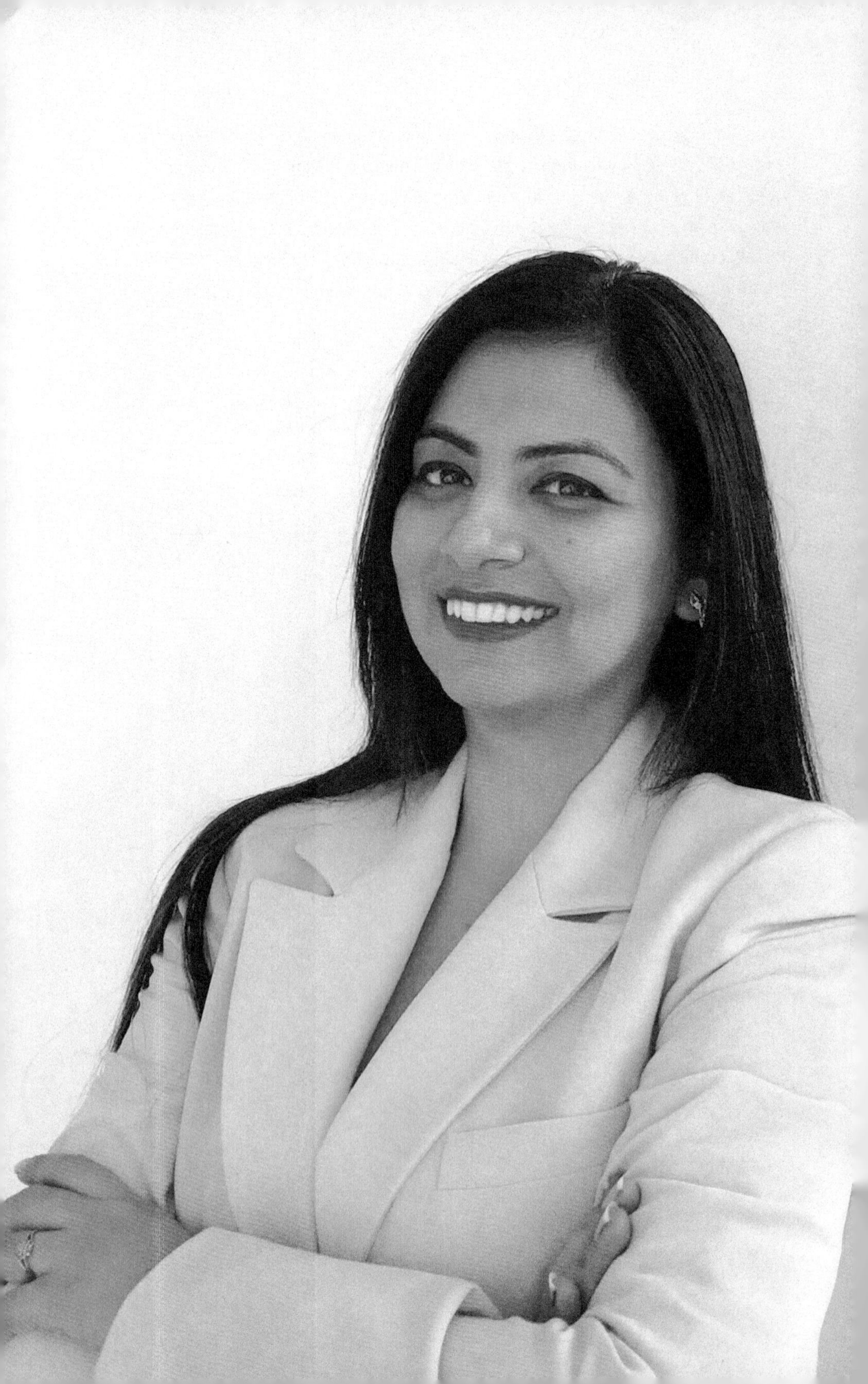

7

RADHIKA BATRA

> ***All my life, I tried to hide my condition from people around me and never talked openly to anyone about it.***

Introduction

I'm Radhika, a 30-year-old female with primary lymphedema on the entire left side of my body, predominantly in the leg, and have lived all my life with this condition. I was born in a small town in Rajasthan, India, and was misdiagnosed for more than 6 years due to a lack of awareness amongst the medical fraternity about lymphedema. Let me briefly take you through my journey with lymphedema and the challenges I handled at different phases of life because I had this condition.

Background & Diagnosis

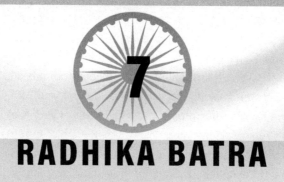

It was the September of 1992 when I was born as a completely healthy child with just a small lump in my groin area. As it is a general Indian practice with new-borns, I was given a few massages and my lump got dissolved so the doctors didn't show any concern. However, when I started walking, the swelling started to develop in my foot, and before we knew it had progressed to my entire leg and the genitals. My parents tried to reach out to doctors to understand what was happening to me, but we hardly got anything but disappointment. It was then we turned towards homeopathy, but the medications prescribed to me were for filariasis and were making me sicker. They did not help with the swelling at all, rather gave me digestion problems, I couldn't eat anything, so we eventually stopped that treatment. By this time I was 5 years old and I hadn't received the right diagnosis, the swelling is getting worse with each passing day. While roaming around the country looking for a diagnosis, we finally came across a physician who referred me to a plastic surgeon in Ahmedabad, which is in the state of Gujrat. This place was nearly 24 hours train journey from my hometown but without thinking twice, we packed our bags and left to meet this surgeon. This was the turning point in my life, and finally, I found a doctor who was certain about what was happening to my body. Looking at my leg, he indicated it could be lymphedema and recommended we visit AIIMS Delhi, a renowned medical research center & hospital in India, and get myself tested for an actual diagnosis. Although he briefly explained lymphedema, there still were many questions, leaving us extremely confused and scared. He advised us to not undertake any surgical treatment until I was an adult. We left that city hopeless yet hopeful, looking forward to finding more answers from AIIMS Delhi. After a struggle of months to get an appointment, I was seen by surgeons at AIIMS. They ordered some tests to confirm my diagnosis, one of them was lymphoscintigraphy, the results of which showed I had insufficient lymph nodes in the left leg and foot for normal lymph circulation while my right leg was completely fine. So, the diagnosis was **Congenital Primary Lymphedema** which is a rare genetic condition, but we were not able to trace anyone in my family to have such a condition.

The diagnosis finally provided some relief as we at least knew what it was. The next obvious step was to find a solution for it, but to our disappointment doctors said there isn't a known cure for it yet, and it can only be managed with compression therapy. I was around 8 years old at that time, and clearly remember that feeling when I heard those doctors talk to my parents telling them that my condition will get worse with time. Our world had just shattered into small pieces at that very moment. Back in the 90s, there were limited resources and not even a handful of lymphedema specialists in a developing country like India. I would say, I got lucky to have met Dr. S.B. Gogia in those days, who specialized in lymphedema and was associated with AIIMS Delhi. He later started his private practice at his own surgical center in Delhi itself.

Lymphedema Journey Begins

When it comes to lymphedema, compression is considered to be one of the most important tools to keep the swelling under control, and that is exactly what I was prescribed. My parents were taught how to bandage me, the skincare, and the precautions to keep infections at bay because with lymphedema one is highly susceptible to them. They learned all about it and took the best care they possibly could. We were in constant touch with Dr. Gogia and would often visit for follow-ups and remeasurements of my leg despite living very far away from him. Although we had some lymphedema management tools, you know how it is with young kids, they are clumsy, always getting dirty while playing, and being trapped in those layers of bandages in India's extremely hot weather, wasn't something I could keep up with. By this time, I was also going to school and becoming more and more cautious about the way I looked and how people would stare at me. We used to have a skirt as part of our school uniform and I hated wearing skirts, as they would draw all the attention to my leg which would lead to a lot of bullying by the kids at school. I remember being called "Elephant legged" and being pushed around to make me fall, and then all of them laughing, making fun of me. Those were some really dark days, but I don't remember coming home sad, complaining about it, or talking to anyone about it. I had somehow accepted being treated like that, which is not really the right thing because, in some way or the other, it was all building up inside me, but I believe it was my way of protecting myself.

Teenage Drama & Challenges

Fast forward a few years to when I was 16 years old. I was consumed by teen-age hormones, not taking care of my leg at all, no bandaging and didn't wear compression for years. One afternoon at school, I felt a slight pain in my little toe, and by evening my entire leg was hurting and I had a very high fever. Even after taking medicine for fever and pain, it wasn't subsiding, I was then rushed to a hospital where they could not diagnose anything for 2 weeks. I was on a pain pump 24/7, and the high dosage of drugs made me hallucinate, but there was no relief from the pain. They were going to discharge me with the diagnosis that I had psychological pain, as all the tests were coming back normal. In the final run of tests before discharge, they found in the MRI that I had some infection in the hip joint because of lymph that had accumulated there, and that was the reason behind the pain. I was then taken for emergency surgery to remove that fluid. The recovery took a month and definitely took its toll on my studies, as I was out of school for 2 months, but finally there was some light at the end of the tunnel. The one major lesson that we learned after going through it all was to consult the lymphedema specialist first whenever anything goes wrong. I feel if I had gone to see Dr Gogia, he would have analysed everything from the Lymphedema angle first.

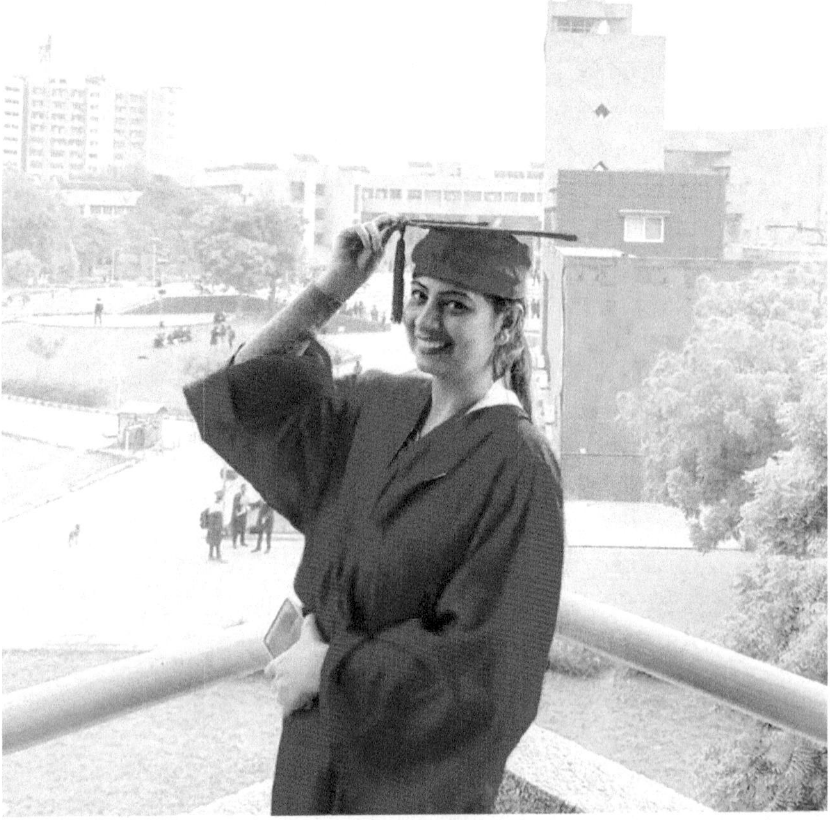

Radhika Batra - Ph.D. Graduation

The next phase of my life started when I moved to Delhi for college. I had made it to one of the top colleges of Delhi University and was going to experience hostel life for the first time. It was scary, exciting and challenging at the same time, since I was so accustomed to special care from my family at home. I was now solely responsible for my lymphedema care, but this did not work out so well. I got so swayed by college life, hectic classes plus lab schedule, self-study time, involvement in various clubs and societies, and all the other chores, my lymphedema care got lost in all that, no matter how much I tried to accommodate it in my routine. I was also angry with myself as a teenager because there were so many things lymphedema would restrict me from doing. I couldn't wear fancy shoes or clothes just like the other college girls and that made me feel inferior. I would hide my swelling under loose clothes and even got trolled and called names for that kind of fashion sense. I remember being heartbroken as I was excluded from participating in the group dance performance because the costume was a short dress. Fortunately, I found a couple of friends who always stood by me and helped me sail through those tough times. They were the angels God sent to protect me.

I graduated with honors and went ahead to pursue higher studies at IIT Delhi. Everything went smoothly for the first couple of months, until suddenly one day I felt severe pain in the lymphedema leg. Without hesitation I went to see my lymphedema specialist, after all, one of the main reasons to continue education in Delhi was to have access to emergency care. He scolded me first for ignoring my leg as the swelling had reached its worst state. It was so hard and full of lymph, it felt like my leg could burst anytime. I was admitted to his care facility, where I got complete decongestive therapy with 24/7 compression. My pain started to subside within 2-3 days and the swelling went down, dramatically. After a week a lot of fluid had drained out and I had a sack of skin hanging. We then decided to go ahead with a debulking surgery so that I could fit into compression stockings and take better care of myself. My surgery went well, and my leg was smaller than ever. I even started to fit into normal shoes and clothes again! That gave me so much hope and further pushed me to use the compression tools, whatever I had access to. Although I used circular knit compression stockings during the day, a compression pump and bandages at night, my swelling still couldn't retain the post-surgery state. However, despite all the struggles, I not only managed to get my master's degree but also decided to continue with a Ph.D. in the next couple of years. I did not want lymphedema to limit my life and even though I had to spend long-standing hours in the lab for my research work, I gathered the strength to carry on and earned a doctorate in chemistry. Along with these academic triumphs, I also followed my passion for dancing and different adventurous activities like hiking, river rafting and paragliding.

My Personal Awakening

All my life, I tried to hide my condition from people around me and never talked openly to anyone about it, which resulted in a lot of emotional baggage and made me feel empty inside. After almost 3 years of my surgery, one fine evening, I decided to go vocal about it. I started looking for people with lymphedema on social media and was stunned by so many lovely lymphies on Instagram. I created a new account with the Instagram handle **indian_lymphie**, took a picture of my lymphie leg, and posted it. I was so overwhelmed by all the love people poured into that picture. That gave me more courage to talk about it openly. I started sharing everything on that account including my personal hacks, lows & highs with lymphedema, struggles and suggestions, emotional outbursts, everything! It became one of the mediums for me to even spread awareness about lymphedema. It gives me a sense of contentment when I receive messages from people from different parts of the world, even from India, saying I motivate them, and they find my page beneficial for tackling lymphedema and its consequences.

The lymphedema community on Instagram helped me so much when I moved to Canada last year. A friend I made on Instagram referred me to my current Lymphedema therapist, Alla Hardoon. She is such a gem of a person! She has been my saviour all this time in Canada. She helped me access the right compression garments, connected me with the right doctors, and even guided me to get covered under the provincial health insurance benefits plan. I reduced my leg size within 3 weeks by using flat-knit compression stockings, she suggested I use. Now that most management tools are easily accessible to me, it is less challenging to live with this condition.

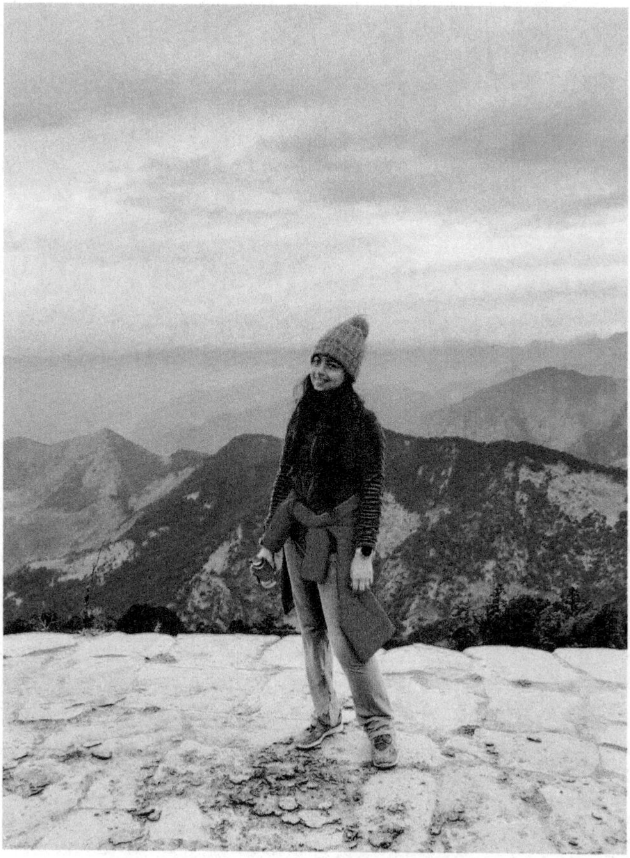

Radhika Batra - My last hiking trip

TOP TIP!

Don't abandon your lymphedema. Take a break if you need to but don't ignore it completely. It is a physically and emotionally consuming condition but turning a blind eye to it will only make things worse.

sigvaris

Reclaim your independence with wraps

Sigvaris wraps are premium garments with innovative designs to accommodate various disease states and improve quality of life.

The Compreflex line offers eight products for all body zones (foot, calf, knee, thigh, arm) and provides accurate, measured compression for self-managed care.

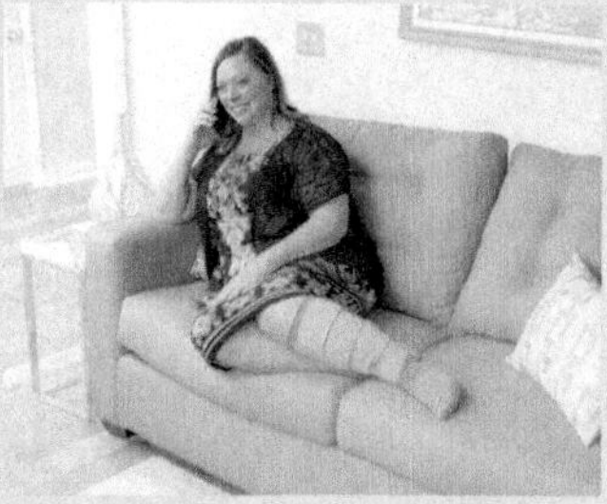

Sigvaris Compreflex

The three Coolflex products (foot, calf, arm) are lightweight garments designed with accurate, measured compression. Their unique Spacer Fabric transfers almost 60% more vapor away from the skin when compared to traditional compression materials. They keep the skin cool and dry to aid with comfort, their double layer design allows for airflow and hook comfort.

Why choose Sigvaris wraps?

- Adaptive size for all volumes foster self-management and empowerment
- The Coolflex range allows one-hand donning, thus promoting even more independence
- Less expensive and obtrusive, more comfortable and hygienic than bandages

Live your life. Be yourself. With flat knit products OPTIFORM

Sigvaris flat knit compression garments meet the requirements of wearers who expect more than mere functionality and effectiveness from their chosen product. Numerous model variants for all body parts and additional options are available for this purpose.

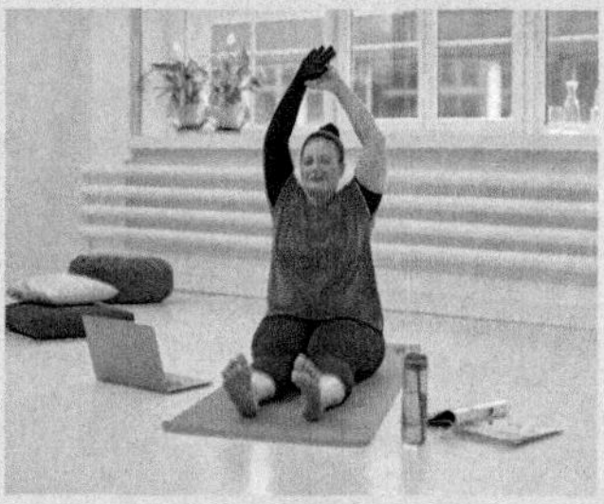

Sigvaris OPTIFORM

All products live up to the promise of their name, Optiform: They offer best support and stabiliity as well as maximum wearing comfort due to their unique manufacturing technology and fiber composition.

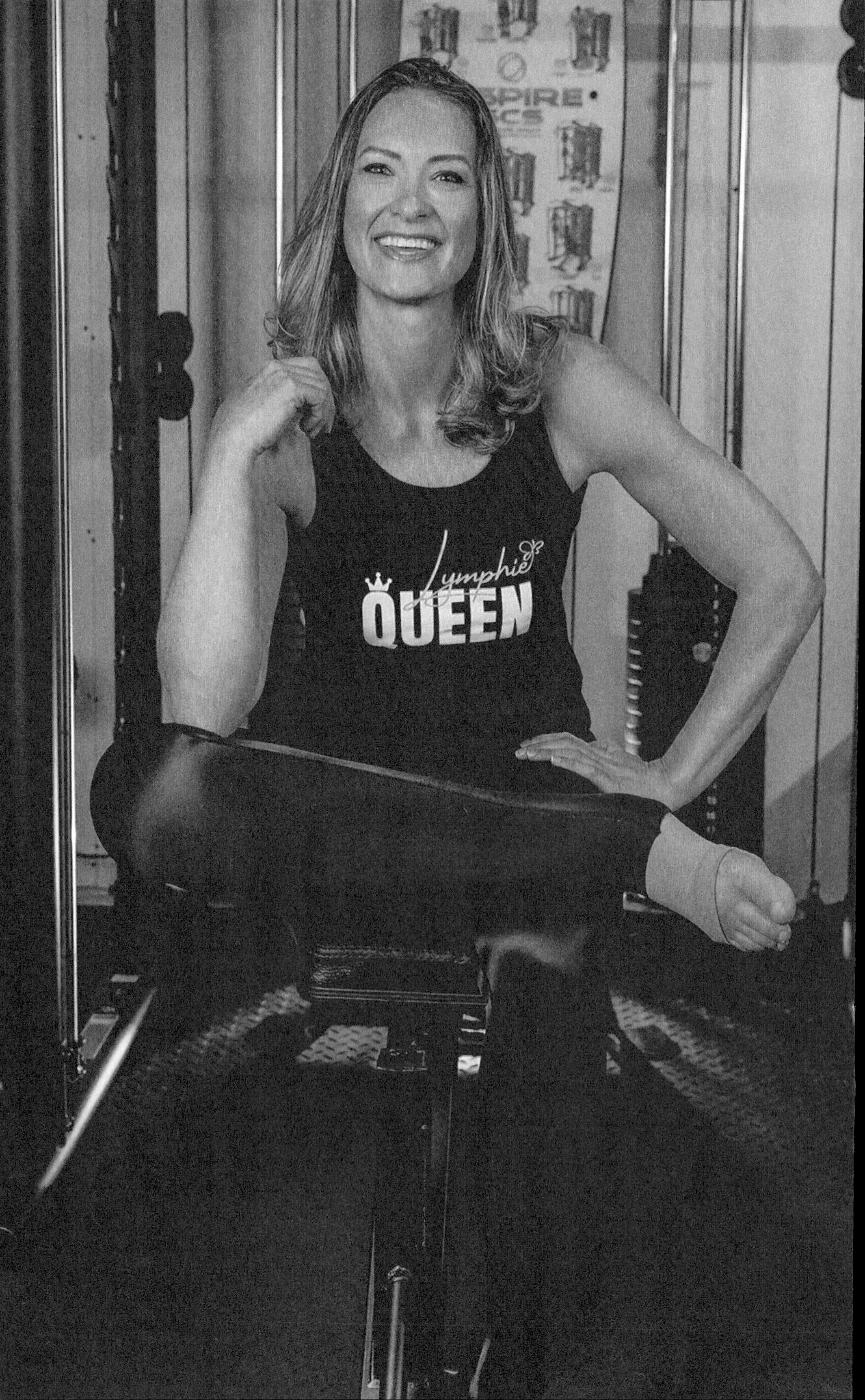
Lymphie
QUEEN

8

AMANDA SOBEY

> ***It was now clear to me that a could not pretend my illness didn't exist. I had to learn to live with it.***

Lymphedema is a disease that appears to still not be well understood by professionals in the medical system. The cause of my Lymphedema is still a mystery to me and learning how to manage the disease has been a long journey. Initially being diagnosed with Lymphedema can be a traumatizing experience, it took me several years to come to terms with my condition. In time, I transformed my attitude from denial and recklessness to acceptance and commitment.

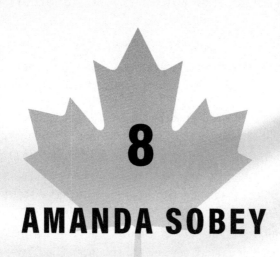

I grew up in Winnipeg and at the age of twenty I made the choice to move to Vancouver and try my luck in the big city. I quickly picked up a job as a cocktail waitress at a posh lounge in Kitsilano. My lifestyle changed rapidly, between making excellent money in tips (for a twenty-year-old) and rolling out in a fast-paced big city, life was truly exciting for me. I spent my time rolling blading along the ocean boardwalks, perusing through local produce at the outdoor markets and enjoying the many nightclubs around the city. After nearly a year of living in Vancouver I experienced a few situations that I believe may have contributed to my diagnosis, they occurred during one week that I will never forget.

I was at the beach when a mosquito bit me, the bite quickly swelled up but it was not itchy, it was hot and peculiar. I didn't think much of it in the days to follow and continued with my usual routines. Friday rolled around and I got invited to a nightclub with some girls I had recently met. Keen to build a social network, I got myself prettied up and hit the town! The club wasn't exactly a wholesome environment, so I decided to linger for a bit, and hit the dance floor. Out of nowhere several women that I did not know began to attack me. Out of shock I covered my head and ran directly into the bouncer. I had never experienced such violence in my life.

I needed to nurse my wounds, but I noticed that my foot began to swell rapidly before my eyes, it became balloon looking. My doctor referred me to a specialist. Meantime, the swelling in my foot began to spread up to my ankle, a few weeks later up to my calf and after one month my entire right leg was filled. At the specialist's office, I underwent a lymphoscintigraphy test. The pain was agonizing as the doctor injected serum between my swollen toes. Once the results came in, he said "your lymphatic system is compromised". He continued to inform me that the condition was known as Secondary Lymphedema (LE). In a short-lowered voice, he said that there was no cure for my condition and that I would need Manual Lymphatic Drainage (MLD) once a week for the rest of my life. He handed me a prescription for compression stockings and swiftly walked out of the room.

I could not believe what I had just been told. I thought that I was going to a specialist to fix my leg and was left feeling scarred for life. After taking time off work in order to recover, I began to feel disconnected from everyone and none of my young new friends could provide the support I needed to snap out of that mindset. Over the following four months I lived in complete denial. I began to self-medicate with alcohol, it helped me to detach from the reality that my leg was completely engorged and puffy like memory foam. I wanted to believe that it was all a mistake and that I would wake up one morning and the condition would disappear as fast as it came.

One day for no apparent reason I decided to purchase my compression stockings, it took some trial and error but once I found the right fit, I regretted waiting so long. Sampling the different makes and models of LE garments was a critical step in my satisfaction with them. Some garments would bunch behind my knee causing painful heat pimples, while other garments would have a silicone band at the top that would fold and pinch in my groin area. Once I found the right brand it was like a dream, and I wore them as consistently as possible. There were times I had a cellulitis infection when they were impossible to wear but I did the best I could.

Over the following year I continuously obsessed about my condition. It affected me daily, especially my wardrobe. As a cocktail waitress image played a large part in my success, in the past my attire included skirts and high heels. The pressure to dress hypersexual while pretending to be at ease in this industry is immense. Attempting to factor into my outfits a swollen leg and foot compounded the pressure and humiliation, it left me feeling deformed and ugly. I tried to hide it, but the eight hours of discomfort and pain was unbearable. I could no longer do my job; my self-confidence was lost. I quit serving and got a part-time job as a receptionist, it was now clear to me that a could not pretend my illness didn't exist. I had to learn to live with it.

It took several more months before I finally decided to try Manual Lymphatic Drainage (MLD). Just like my experience with the compression, finding the right massage or physiotherapist took some time. The experience was very personal for me, the first few therapists I tried left me feeling unsatisfied and without medical insurance I was quick to give up on the whole idea. After a few more months my body was telling me I needed something more than just the garments, so I committed myself to finding a therapist that had experience with lymphatic drainage and someone

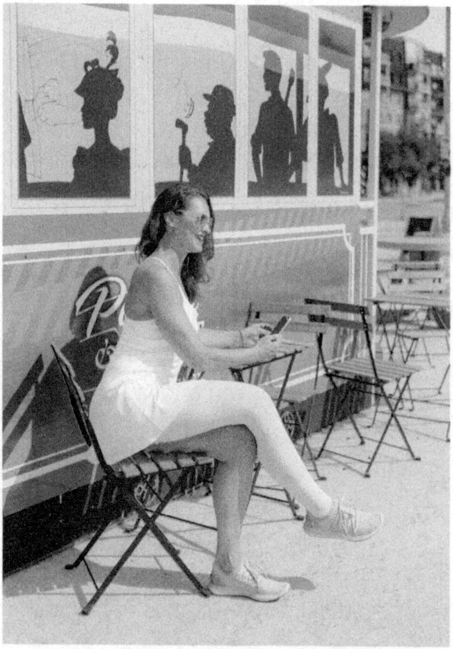

Amanda Sobey outside café

I felt comfortable with. Finally, the fourth therapist I tried worked for me but she was located in Winnipeg so I couldn't always get the service I needed but at the very least I knew that MLD was effective, I just didn't have good access to it.

I felt completely vulnerable to my condition and remained straddled with low self-regard, but life goes on and over the next few years I married and had two children. My first pregnancy triggered a wave of urgency for me. I knew I needed to manage my overall health for the betterment of my child and keeping my swelling and fluid retention at bay throughout the pregnancy. I began to exercise regularly and turned my attention towards nutrition. The cleaner the diet and regular exercise helped me to cope well with the excess fluid however, after the baby was born my skin grew increasingly firm and it became more difficult to reduce the swelling. I believe that I was exhibiting signs of Stage II Lymphedema.

Just over a year later I became pregnant with my second child. With a demanding infant on hand, coupled with prolonged sleepless nights I was too exhausted to maintain the same health standards this time around. After a long pregnancy, the baby was born colicky and now I had two infants to care for with a husband that worked out of town more than three-quarters of the time. Still relatively new to Vancouver, there were few people I could turn to for any sort of respite. My family loved me from afar, but I had to cope with a lot on my own. Always putting myself second threw me into a perpetual state of strain.

Meanwhile my marriage was deteriorating rapidly, everything that could have gone wrong between two people did. After 5 years of hardship and isolation the only thing I could do was to pack up my young children and move back to my hometown. In Winnipeg, my family graciously helped me with the necessities of life, but it was subtly apparent that our connection was different, after all they had lived their day-to-day lives without me for several years. Similar to my family, old friends had moved on with their busy lives, in small ways I was pieced into my old social network but overall, I was starting over. Without reliable childcare, meeting other parents and securing full-time employment was a long struggle. My LE remained symptomatic at Stage II and my coping skills for life in general were depleting. The beginning stages of depression began to set in.

After a difficult year of transition, I began to address my health again. I tried the elimination diet, running, swimming, soccer, MLD and hot/cold therapy to name a few. Regardless of my efforts, in 2010 my leg was at its fullest and heaviest to-date. For two full years I gave up hope for any improvement in my health. By 2012 I had enough. I was willing to try anything, and I did. Around my busy parenting schedule, I got back on track with my MLD therapist, used a compression pump, a micro-current machine, the inversion table, a poultice, reflexology, cold baths, various skin oils and exfoliants and even a rolling pin! I knew compression was effective, so I focused on perfecting the products and my techniques. I purchased four individual stockings and a set of bandages for wrapping and committed to wearing my stockings every day and began wrapping my whole leg at night. The endeavour was exhausting and financially draining however, it did stabilize my symptoms, but nothing seemed to truly reduce my LE.

When I finally secured full-time work that was compatible with my childcare commitments, I was ready to give it my all. I worked tirelessly for eight-hour shifts, got home to manage household chores, tended to the children's education, extracurricular and health needs. On top of that I fiercely carved out time to maintain my LE care regime. It was the same routine everyday non-stop until the minute my head hit the pillow. Finding time for something as little as a haircut took careful planning at least three weeks in advance. After one year, the non-stop circuit was taking its toll on my body. I noticed that my mobility was becoming impaired, and my skin was hardening and appeared to be buckling under the heaviness of my leg. I was exhibiting symptoms of stage III LE. My vision to be healthy and all of my efforts were for nothing! I had lost hope, depression tightened its grip on me, I lost my job and became bed ridden for months to follow.

At that moment, the combination of my physical and mental health could have easily hospitalized me or ended my life. I looked over at my kids, they needed me. I needed a mental shift. It took all of my brain power to convince myself that the hard times have come to pass, and the reality is that success requires trial and error. I began to research my condition further and started with small, manageable changes. Firstly, I committed to drinking more water. Second, I made a list of all the foods that worsened my condition. My list was long and included things like bagels, deep fried foods, Chinese food and potato chips. After analyzing what I ate, I decided to analyze how I eat. By studying and understanding the chemical compositions of food, it became clear that balancing my macronutrients was a game changer. Lastly, I revamped my fitness plan and improved my technique! Every day my physical and emotional health began to recover a little more. I will never forget the day while I was outside with my son fundraising. I felt a warm wind blowing through my pant leg, it had been over a decade since I felt my pants loose around my leg. I will never forget that day.

Out of all of the treatments I had tried over the years I finally figured out what really worked for me, a daily routine. My routine consisted of exercise, anti-inflammatory diet, compression garments, compression wraps, MLD, skincare, and one critical component that I had overlooked until recently -stress management.

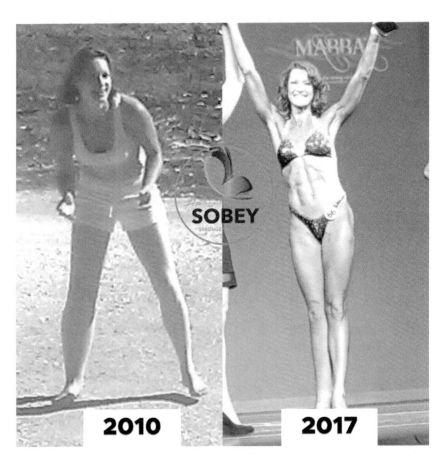

Amanda Sobey - Before and after

Bit by bit, all my hard work was starting to pay off. On October 21, 2017, I reached a personal best when I entered myself into an All-Natural Bodybuilding Competition-Figure Category. I entered the competition for a couple reasons. The first reason was one of my girlfriends told me that I should. Secondly, I felt it was a good goal for someone like me who has been physically disfigured, to compete in an industry where they judge you on symmetry. To my disbelief, the judges did not notice my "bad" leg. I placed 1st and 3rd that day. Since then, I have competed multiple times and can honestly say that body building is a true passion of mine.

Through my own personal trials of health and wellness, I have managed to significantly reduce my edema and improve my mental health through exercise, nutrition, and self-care. I am proud to be the president for the Lymphedema Association of Manitoba helping to create awareness and advocacy. Professionally, I am a Certified Personal Trainer, Certified Nutritionist, and Lymphie Coach. I specialize in helping others with Lymphedema, Lipedema, and Lipolymphedema. I love to help others easily and safely overcome their health struggles as I truly believe we are stronger together.

To learn more about me and the work I do to help those dealing with lymphedema, visit my website www.amandasobey.com. Please feel free to like, follow and share: Facebook: @am.sobey Instagram: @am.sobey LinkedIn: @am-sobey YouTube: @AmandaSobey

TOP TIP!

If I had one piece of advice, it would be to transform your mindset and your attitude.

"Whether you think you can, or think you can't, you're right."

—HENRY FORD

This disease does not define you.

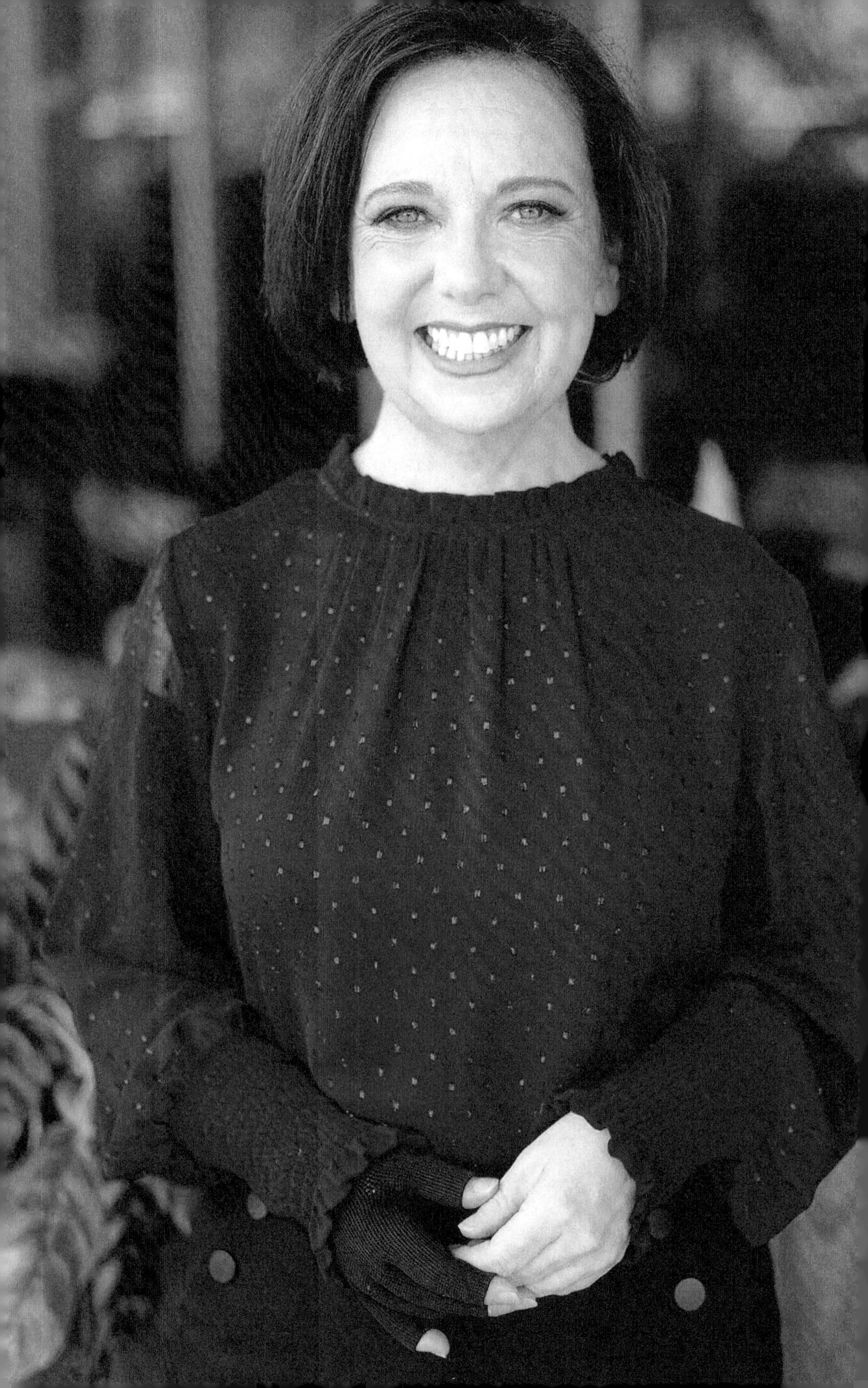

9

MONIQUE BAREHAM

> *Lymphoedema has given me a sense of purpose I could never have imagined.*

My first memory of lymphoedema is when I was being prepared for intensive cancer treatment. It was 2009, I was 37, fit, and apart from my cancer, I was healthy. I was handed a photocopy of arm exercises and told, "You won't get lymphoedema. Only old fat women get lymphoedema."

Less than two months later I was diagnosed with severe early stage lymphoedema. Just like that, I entered what I later called the 'Lymphoedema Maze.'

Despite Cancer Treatment Related Lymphoedema (CTRL) being a known side effect of my treatment, it still took several expensive specialist appointments, misinformation, and a misdiagnosis before I was accurately diagnosed.

I found my lymphoedema diagnosis more devastating than my cancer diagnosis. I was shocked and I felt I had somehow failed. Despite all the arm exercises, my symptoms worsened. When the most invasive parts of my treatment concluded, I sought health advice and was told "You should just be thankful to have survived cancer and only had 'this' to deal with." In comparison to the supportive wrap-around cancer care I was receiving, my lymphoedema care experience felt like falling into an abyss.

This is a life changing, progressive, incurable chronic condition. The pictures I saw on Dr Google were frightening.

This led to my early retirement as I was deemed unfit for duty and placed on a pension.

This was expensive. The crippling cost of compression garments and private specialists combined with the financial toxicity of cancer treatment saw me take a deep dive into financial distress.

This could make me incredibly sick with cellulitis leaving me too scared to pat my cat, garden, exercise or fly in case I ended up in hospital.

This negatively affected my body image. It prompted stares and questions from strangers and triggered feelings of grief every day I wore my ugly, ill fitted, worn out garments.

This made me feel so lonely, isolated and depressed that I imagined an arm amputation would be a better option and questioned the point of surviving cancer.

I sank into despair, truly believing I was the only person my age with lymphoedema. My wakeup call came in the form of three mosquito bites which led to cellulitis. I realised I had to become my own lymphoedema expert fast.

I also needed to find a new life purpose after cancer and its treatments had taken everything I understood about life away from me. I knew I wanted to give back and I saw gaps everywhere, but I couldn't see a place for me to contribute.

The journey of 1000 miles begins with a single step.

I wish I could say I linked in with others who understood my fears and provided peer support, but this was not the case. It was the early days of social media so online support pages and groups were few. I certainly did not find one for lymphoedema.

Eventually, I stumbled across the Lymphoedema Support Group of South Australia (LSGSA) created by motivated lymphoedema patients in 1991. Sadly, by the time I reached out in 2012 it was close to folding. To my dismay, none of the small group left holding the fort had lived experience or clinical knowledge. I appreciated the good intentions, but I came away feeling worse. A few months later, I had no other option, so I gave them a second go as this time there were two guest speakers, Professor Neil Piller, Director of the Flinders University Lymphoedema Clinical Research Unit and a Lymphology PhD candidate, Dr Malou van Zanten.

This was a turning point because as I sat in the front row of a drab, cold Church Hall sipping terrible coffee, I madly scribbled notes as light bulbs started switching on in my head. Finally, I had found two lymphoedema experts who really cared, and they were right on my doorstep! Suddenly I no longer felt alone.

I mulled over this for several months and concluded that the area of greatest need where I could affect change was in lymphoedema. I realised I had found my new purpose; I would be a Lymphoedema Patient Advocate!

Then I had to work out how because there was no roadmap!

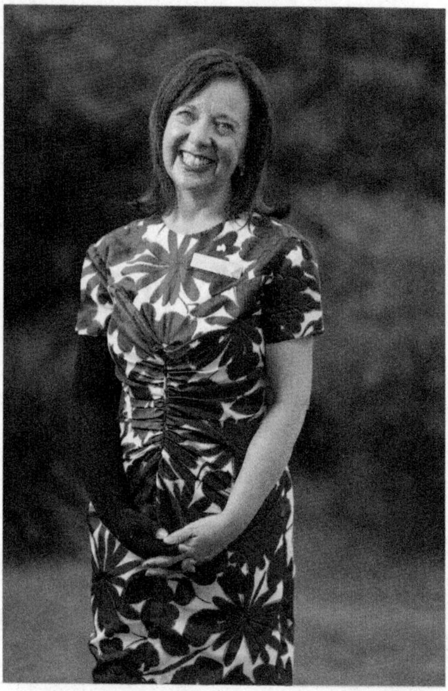

Monique Bareham wearing Compression Sleeve

Lymph-O-What?

I found out quickly that lymphoedema was under-recognised across Australia and internationally. Then I learned that South Australia was the only state in Australia without a compression garment subsidy. I was appalled. I began devising a plan, my first action item was to join the LSGSA committee. Then I wanted to learn as much as I could, so I registered to participate in clinical trials at the Flinders University Lymphoedema Clinical Research Unit.

Within months Prof. Piller invited me to participate in the first of what became many, free lymphoedema information and screening sessions with his team which included visiting rural and regional areas of South Australia. Not only did I learn about the lymphatic system and lymphatic disorders, I learned what gold standard lymphoedema care actually looked like. Dr van Zanten taught me self-management techniques and how to prepare and recover from lengthy road travel and flights.

These trips brought me face-to-face with some of the most vulnerable and neglected individuals affected by lymphoedema in South Australia. I met individuals living with lymphoedema, I met their loved ones, and I met the nurses left to fill the gaps in care. Every place I looked I saw problems with access to affordable specialist lymphoedema care and garments. I found this extremely confronting at first, but as I listened to each heart-breaking story and saw the personal impact and needless suffering caused by long term unmanaged lymphoedema, I became more determined to step up and face this challenge.

In 2013 I became President of the LSGSA (now LASA – Lymphoedema Association of South Australia) and totally reinvigorated it. I created the three Foundational Pillars: Peer Support, Empowerment and Advocacy and introduced the Lymphoedema Patient Advocate role. I found recruiting and maintaining volunteer committee members challenging and exhausting, but, by 2015, LSGSA had become a trusted source of reliable information and peer support. I felt I was now ready to start some serious advocating.

Lymphoedema is a hard sell. It is under-diagnosed and just not 'sexy.' Crucially, lymphoedema is not recorded in Australian health statistics so it is so difficult to make a case or attract and maintain media interest. This meant I had to be creative, reliable, and respectfully persistent.

In the lead up to March 2015, while on break, I began thinking about how I could raise awareness during Lymphoedema Awareness Month. I had just set up my new lymphoedema advocacy Facebook page and I was keen to create an online campaign. I decided to post a daily fact about lymphoedema and tie it to the message: South Australia is the only state without a lymphoedema compression garment subsidy scheme. To my surprise, it really took off across Australia and Internationally, what was to be a quiet month suddenly became incredibly hectic. With the help of Dr van Zanten, I sourced and wrote a new evidence based lymphoedema fact every day for 31 days in a row.

It is vitally important to me that I remain connected with other individuals affected by lymphoedema. I always learn new things and it enables me to remain an effective voice for change. I spend hours making calls, having Zoom meetings and writing emails to other 'lymphies' Australia wide. I often joke that much of my work happens from my bed, in my pyjamas with my cat, Mr Lincoln, by my side.

Before COVID-19, I attended countless face-to-face coffee catch ups, which is quite a feat in itself given South Australia spreads across 983,482 km^2 and is about five times the size of the UK. I have lost count of the hours and kilometres I have racked up on the road between my home in metropolitan Adelaide and Mt Gambier, six hours away in the South East or seven hours up and over Spencer Gulf to Port Lincoln on the Lower Eyre Peninsula.

One notable breakthrough happened quite suddenly following a late afternoon phone message from a rural patient group. The Federal Minister for Health would be attending a community forum the next day! I immediately dropped what I was doing, asked the ladies to meet me at the hall, called the office of the Local Member and drove six hours to be there. Within 24 hours, I was standing with the local support group speaking with the Federal Minister for Health.

Slowly I started to see change happening. Members of Parliament attended LSGSA events and Cancer Council SA was supporting us. Our information sessions were regularly attracting 50-plus participants and brought together consumers, therapists, researchers and industry representatives from South Australia and interstate.

In 2019, I was invited to become a member of the first South Australian Lymphoedema Advisory Group. In July 2020, and in the middle of the COVID-19 Pandemic, my advocacy led to the launch of the first South Australian Lymphoedema Compression Garment Subsidy Scheme. It was a remarkable and satisfying step forward.

However, my advocacy also called for the development of affordable lymphoedema clinics. Without them, many of our most vulnerable could not access the scheme. In September 2020, I proudly spent my 49th birthday socially distanced and in a mask with physiotherapists and registered nurses, Prof. Piller and others participating in the first SA Health compression garment training session. This was the first step toward establishing public lymphoedema care in South Australia.

It was a surprise and my honour to receive both the Australian of the Year's, 2022 South Australian Local Hero Award and the Joy Noble Medal in recognition of my volunteer contribution to improving the lives of individuals affected by lymphoedema. I am truly humbled. But the most exciting part for me, is the recognition they have brought to lymphoedema and the scope they give me to advocate further. I know the issues do not stop at the South Australian border, so I grabbed the opportunity to shine a light on lymphoedema with both hands! My dream is to see every individual across Australia affected by lymphoedema counted in Australian health data and able to access affordable, evidence-based care and garments.

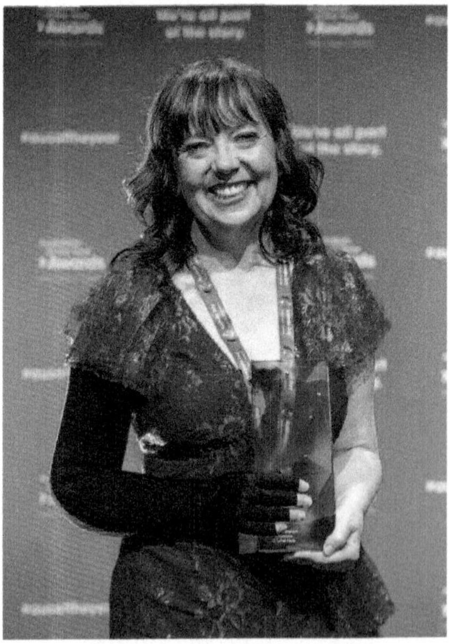

Monique Bareham - SA Australian of the Year Award 2021

I used the platform my role of South Australian Local Hero 2022 provided to raise the lack of data on the prevalence of lymphoedema in Australia. This led to an invitation to contribute to the first Australian Institute of Health and Welfare (AIHW) report on lymphoedema. I am excited to share that the report titled, 'Toward an estimate of the prevalence of lymphoedema in Australia' was released on June 20 2023. As the only dedicated lymphoedema patient advocate included, I welcome this progress and look forward to contributing to future analytical reports describing the prevalence of lymphoedema in Australia.

I am currently working with Ms Louise Miller-Frost MP, Federal Member for Boothby and Dr Monique Ryan MP, Federal Member for Kooyong on preparations for the imminent launch of the first Australian Parliamentary Friends of Lymphoedema Group.

I didn't know it at the time, but my lymphoedema diagnosis was to become the single most important and transformative event in my life. Lymphoedema has given me a sense of purpose I could never have imagined. Living with lymphoedema has taught me patience, resilience, and the importance of self-care and through my lymphoedema I have met inspiring and kind individuals who I am privileged to call friends. Lymphoedema reminds me of the wise words of Alanis Morissette, "Life has a funny way of helping you out". Isn't that ironic.

TOP TIP!

Listen to your body, it can send you a signal something's not right. If you act on it quickly, you may dodge the problem.

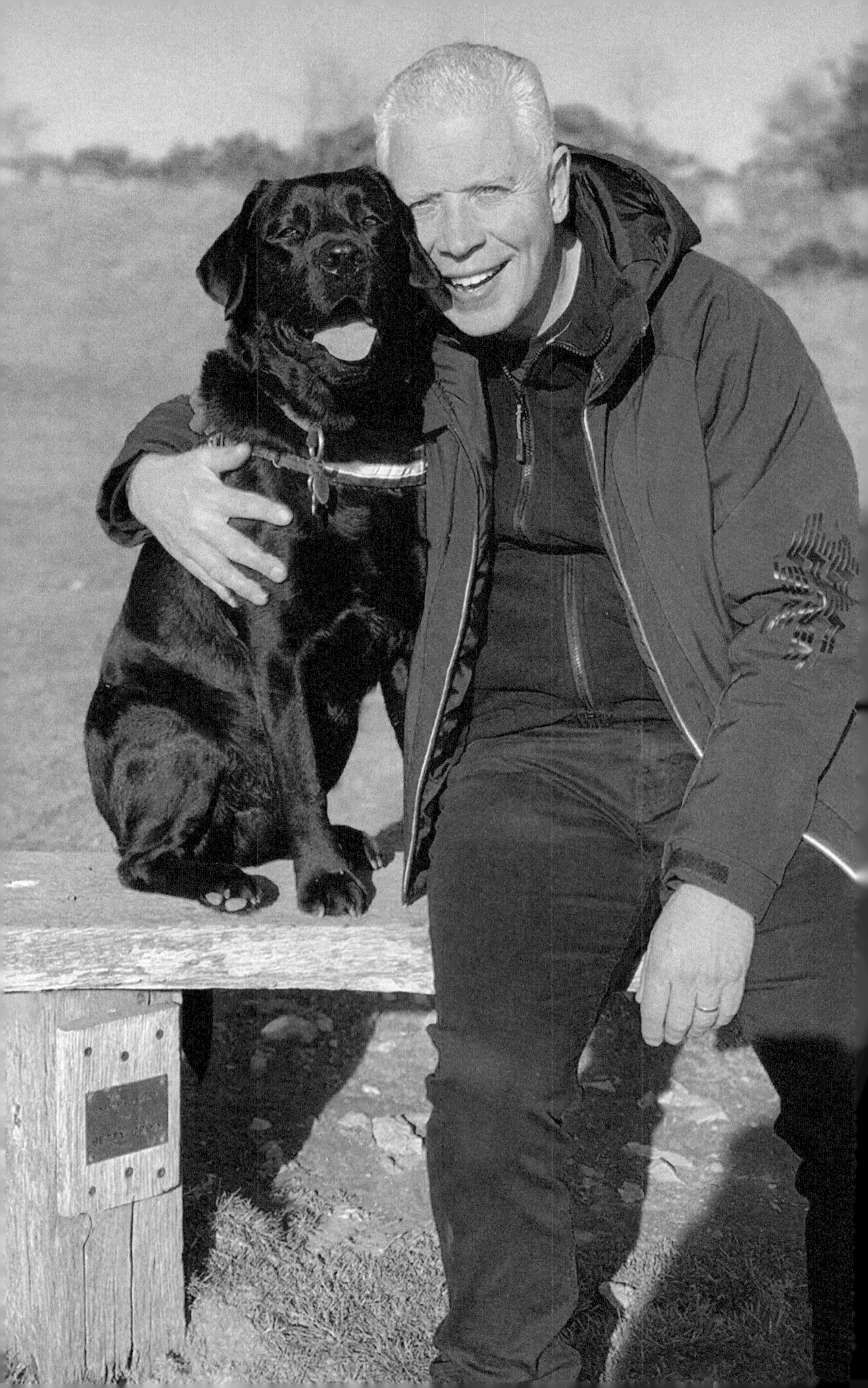

10

GRAHAM ROOMS

> ***She warned me this would leave me with lifelong conditions such as incontinence and erectile dysfunction, but at no stage was lymphoedema ever mentioned.***

My lymphoedema journey started in December 2019 shortly after having surgery for aggressive prostate cancer. Before surgery my consultant had told me she was going to carry out a non-nerving sparing procedure which included the removal of inguinal lymph nodes. She warned me this would leave me with lifelong conditions such as incontinence and erectile dysfunction, but at no stage was lymphoedema ever mentioned.

It was at my 6-week post-surgery meeting when I mentioned I was experiencing a slight swelling in the right side of my pubic area. I believed it was simply surgical scaring which would go down after a while, but after a brief examination she stated it could be lymphoedema and she would refer me to the local team.

I wasn't overly worried, after all it was the cancer, I wanted to get rid of and anything that came about as a consequence of the surgery was insignificant in comparison. Like most people, I didn't really know what lymphoedema was and believed it was just a temporary condition.... how wrong I was!

After meeting with my local lymphoedema team they marked up my legs to take measurements and advised me on some basic massage methods using a mini paint roller. It was all very antiquated and provided little insight into what was to come. Even after my initial consultation I still didn't comprehend the significance of my condition as my focus was still very much on my cancer and I was relieved that early tests were showing positive outcomes. I was prescribed a pair of compression pants that I was instructed to wear daily to help manage the swelling. I wasn't sure how I could be compliant with wearing these every day as I knew I wouldn't be issued another pair for 6 months.

As my swelling increased and my knowledge of lymphoedema expanded, I started to become very worried about the progressive and chronic nature of the condition and what this meant to me, both physically and mentally. Researching the condition through Dr Google was something I regret as the images that kept appearing were very distressing and disturbing and painted the worst-case scenario.

It was only when I met with my friend Kim that she revealed she also suffered from lymphoedema in her left arm following breast cancer. I often wondered why she wore a sleeve on her arm but had never known or asked why. She advised me to find a therapist who could perform Manual Lymphatic Drainage (MLD) as she had found this very beneficial. After searching for a therapist within my local area I found a lovely lady named Susan who was happy to evaluate my condition. I didn't know then what a saviour Susan would become as there wasn't much she didn't know about the condition.

Over the following weeks I met with Susan on numerous occasions for MLD treatment and she provided guidance on all aspects of self-management, including skin care and compression along with ways to perform manual lymphatic drainage on myself. Sadly, COVID then took over the world and lockdown prevented me visiting for many months. During this period I started to become extremely anxious about my condition and then one day whilst carrying out some DIY I noticed a damp spot on my trousers. I thought I had probably lent against a wet surface but soon realised that wasn't the case. As I took down my trousers, I could see fluid perforating from my skin. I must admit I freaked out and contacted Susan immediately. As always, she provided reassurance and guidance as to what to do. Thankfully the fluid stopped leaking after elevating my leg, but I then experienced another episode weeks later after our pet cat jumped on my leg and clawed my skin. I immediately treated this with antiseptic cream as I had become paranoid about the risk of an infection and cellulitis.

When I look back it was the fluid discharge experiences that really hit home and made me realise I needed to do everything possible to stop my condition worsening. What had started in my pubic area was now clearly in my thighs, and in my mind, it was only a matter of time before it would spread down to my ankles.

During my early MLD sessions with Susan she had used light massage techniques with her hands but then she introduced 'Magic Hands', an electromechanical therapeutic procedure using a deep oscillation machine that creates gentle electrostatic impulses to the skin tissue. As I was unable to see Susan due to COVID I decided to purchase a Deep Oscillation Machine which I could use daily to perform Simple Lymphatic Drainage (SLD) on myself. Although the equipment wasn't cheap it was a beneficial investment whereby, I could partially simulate the MLD treatment that Susan performed on me using a hand applicator. With Susan's help a bespoke 20-minute session was created using high and low frequencies. Each night my bedtime routine consists of pre therapy breathing and hand massage to free up axillary nodes, followed by a deep oscillation session. Life is very different in the bedroom, but my wife and I have adapted to the change with a positive attitude and outlook.

With guidance from Susan, I also developed a meticulous skin care regime which helps with my lymphoedema management. This includes the use of Dermol as a soap substitute, the application of Aveeno After Shower Mist Moisturiser, and Flexitol Heel Balm to prevent blisters or sores developing. For someone who rarely bothered about skin care this is quite a change, but one that is crucial.

Throughout my lymphoedema journey the biggest challenge I have and continue to face is finding a compression garment that can control the swelling in my pubic/genital area. Almost every professional I have met has shared the difficulty of effective compression in this area and my quest for a solution is still ongoing. To date, I have purchased and been issued an array of garments and padding that I have worn during a variety of activities, but sadly I still haven't found anything that has been totally effective. It was this situation along with the fear my condition was worsening that influenced my decision to explore LVA surgery. I had read about this during my early research but as the surgery was quite new and pioneering, I hadn't considered this as an option until now.

After carrying out further research I contacted the Oxford Lymphoedema Practice (OLP) to book an appointment. They are recognised as one of the leading practices in the UK for lymphoedema surgery so I knew I was in the best hands to assess and guide me as to whether this type of surgery would be beneficial. Sadly, the NHS doesn't fund this type of surgery as it is deemed cosmetic. I still fail to understand how a condition caused by cancer surgery is deemed 'cosmetic' which I still argue is discriminatory against lymphoedema sufferers.

My first meeting with the OLP was scheduled for early July 2021 when I met with the consultants to discuss my condition history. Before this I had an MRI scan of my lower limbs which would be used to determine the fat, muscle and fluid composition in my legs. After a lengthy discussion with the consultants (Professor Furniss and Alex Ramsden) my legs were measured using a very sophisticated piece of equipment which was then followed by an ICG lymphography injection in both feet. This injection contained indocyanine green dye which is taken up by the lymphatic and is then visualised using an infra-red camera system.

It was at that moment I realised I could no longer deny my condition as the results were stark and very clear. The camera showed my lymphatics were working as normal up to my knees as there were defined linear pathways, but sadly above the knees was a very different story. Not only was there extensive dermal backflow but also starburst patterns which meant my lymphatic system was struggling to find a pathway.

Professor Furniss described this like a motorway that was blocked by an accident. As cars pass the blocked lanes the traffic flow slows down and drivers attempt to seek alternative routes. In instances where the motorway is blocked completely the traffic comes to a complete standstill with nowhere to go. This is exactly what happens to a damaged lymphatic system whereby pathways become blocked and lymph fluid attempts to find an alternative route. When the lymph fluid comes to a standstill it becomes fibrosis and turns to fat, hence why lymphoedema is termed as a progressive condition. Obviously, the transition from fluid to fat isn't instant, but it all made sense to me and emphasised my precarious and worrying position.

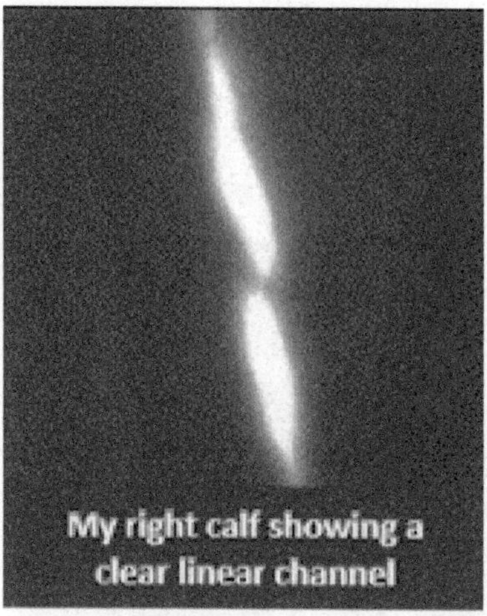

Graham Rooms ICG Results - Right Calf

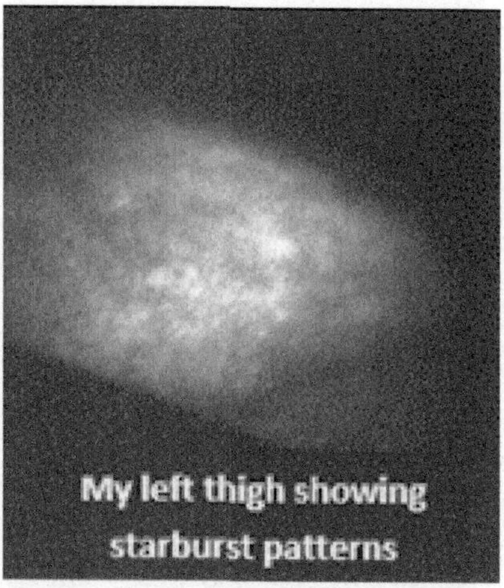

Graham Rooms ICG Results - Left Thigh

Even though the ICG had shown my lymphatics were struggling, Professor Furniss told me I was still a good candidate for LVA surgery due to the staging of my lymphoedema. As with many other conditions early invention provides the best chance of a successful outcome and LVA surgery was no different. The evaluation of success for LVA surgery is based on 3 criteria, an improvement to a patients quality of life (QOL), a reduction in the number of episodes of cellulitis and a reduction in limb size/swelling. Based on the fact I had not had cellulitis and my limb size was not excessive, I knew it would be difficult to evaluate the cost versus benefits

After much deliberation and with the wonderful backing of my wife I decided to go ahead with the surgery. I knew it would be a gamble as there were no guarantees of success, but I asked myself, will this give me the best possible chance of maintaining my mobility and quality of life? Based on everything I had researched and with the professional guidance of Professor Furniss, my answer was an emphatic 'yes.'

The day arrived for my LVA surgery and I woke with a mixture of emotions. Part of me was happy I was doing something positive about my condition, and yet there was still this niggling doubt as to whether the expense of the surgery was something I could justify. I also felt an element of self-pity and anger, thinking why me and why couldn't the NHS fund this as it was caused by my cancer surgery.

As I write this article 18 months after my LVA surgery, I still don't know whether it has totally worked, but as I am still able to get out on the golf course and still have quality of life, in my mind I made the right decision.

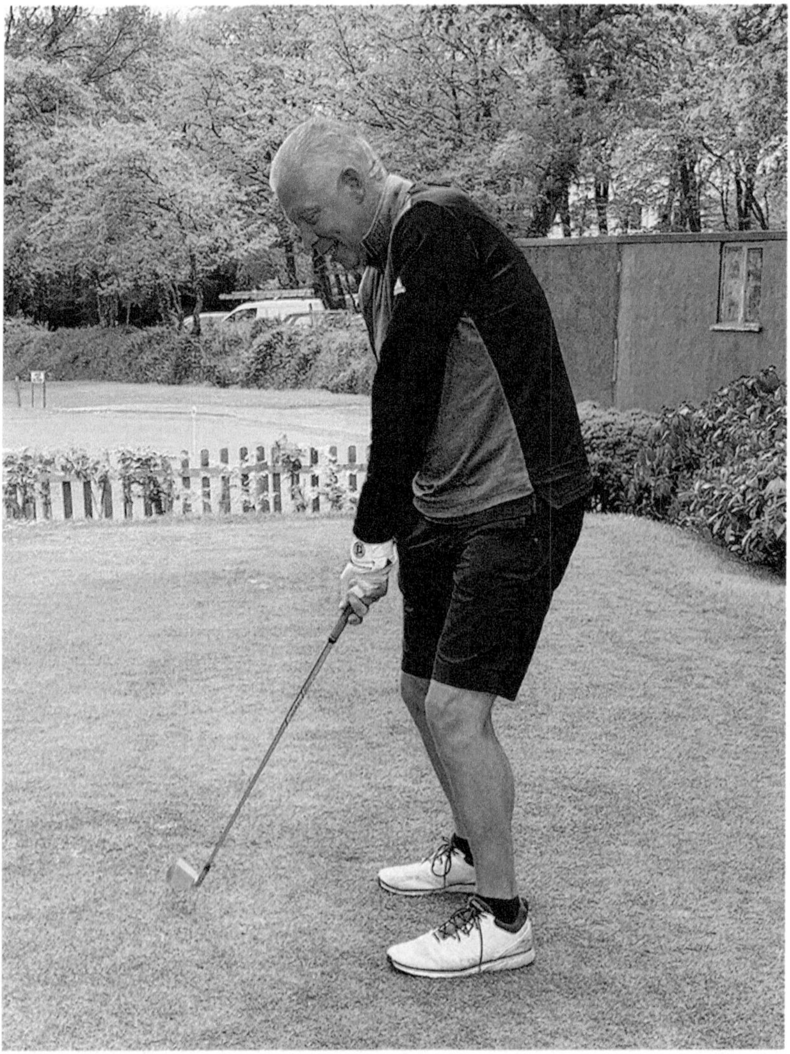

Graham Rooms - FORE!

Even after surgery I still find myself looking for new or alternative treatments which can assist with the management of my lymphoedema. That desire directed me to trying a pneumatic compression pump which I had read about during my early research. Although the equipment isn't cheap, I felt it was a beneficial addition to my lymphoedema management and one that would support me following exercise, which is when I experience the most swelling in my pubic area.

So, there you have my lymphoedema journey to date, which like so many others, includes a mixture of emotions and frustrations. Whilst lymphoedema remains so underfunded by the NHS we will continue to see the post code lottery of treatment and care. Thankfully, there are now some fantastic groups for sufferers such as Lymphoedema United who are sharing experiences and spreading the word about effective garments and solutions.

Whilst my lymphoedema journey will be forever, I do feel content that I have done everything possible to stop a deterioration of my condition and given myself the best chance of maintaining my quality of life, which is vital for my mental health and general wellbeing.

TOP TIP!

Push hard to get the best treatment and support possible, along with a robust self-care routine. This is the best combination to stop the progression of this debilitating condition.

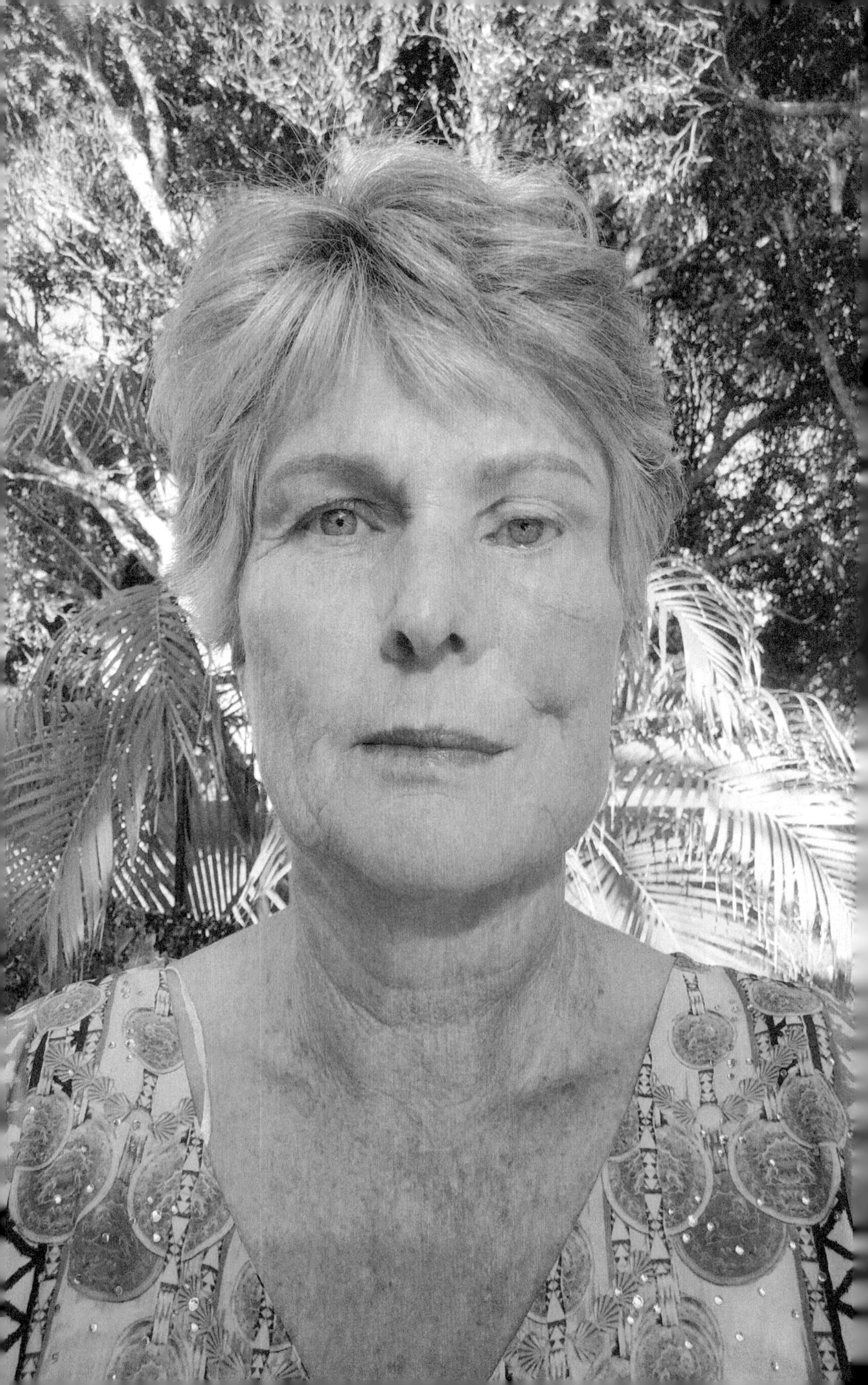

11

HELEN MACLEAN

> ***I still enjoy all my outdoor pursuits.***
> ***Oh, to smile for a day.***

My name is Helen and I live in New Zealand. I've been treated for cancer to the trigeminal nerve, undergoing a 12-hour surgery, chemo, and 6 weeks of intensive radiotherapy all during the Covid-19 lockdowns, and I am dyslexic. So, I chose to spend time writing about my story because I feel very strongly in sharing and helping others on this journey.

Where to start. It took two and a half years to get diagnosed with squamous cell cancer to the right trigeminal nerve. This is one of the cranial nerves in the head and is responsible for providing sensation and movement to the face. One nerve runs to the right side of the head, the other to the left. Although hard to diagnose this was not surprising and somewhat frustrating for me due to my family history which was all revealed to my GP's (General Practitioners). A Father with the same cancer but not including the trigeminal nerve, a mother with breast cancer, sister with ovarian cancer and, a second sister with non-Hodgkin's lymphoma cancer. "HELLO..."

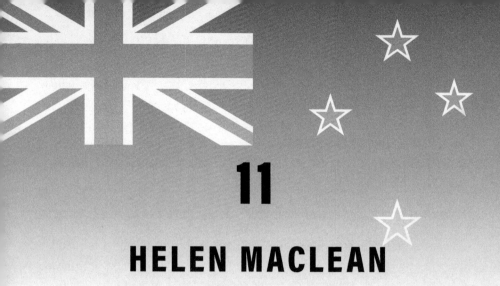

Long story short, I was on my third GP who told me, "Helen, at your age, (late 50's) you must expect some aches and pains". Hence my trip to ER and pleading with the doctor not to release me without finding a problem. She tried her hardest but with no result, "God bless her soul" she referred me to a private neurologist. Many scans later he saw the problem and referred me to a surgeon. "Happy days, I had a diagnosis".

Note to self, getting cancer in the first lockdowns of a global pandemic is not ideal.

Before we go any further, who am I? Wife of 37 years, meeting my husband through a mutual love of skydiving. Mother to two adult girls, with two beautiful granddaughters. My youngest daughter was diagnosed with Crohn's disease aged 6 years old and I soon learnt how to navigate the health system through her. Before Covid I was running a small B&B and tutoring dyslexic students. "Tutoring?", I hear you query! I addressed my own dyslexia in my 40's, unlocking the joy and thrill of learning. I did some study and now get to share the learning. I'm an active relaxer. I cycle, paddle board, wave ski, boating, fishing, and travel, even though it's a "bit of a trek" to live down under.

How to navigate the National Health System, while calling on the back up of health insurance and personal funds? Don't think for a moment that my husband and I are moneyed. At the time he was a firefighter and I worked part time, self-employed.

While being diagnosed as a private patient it soon became clear that treatments would well exceed my insurance policy. My surgeon was brilliant and jumped me back into the National Health System for my surgery. With the money saved I was able to convince my insurance company to pay for the radiotherapy, but I needed to fund the Chemo myself. This three-way split has been an ongoing necessity during my two years of treatments, striving to facilitate good outcomes. "Yes, I'm worth It".

Now here's where I revert to bullet points:

- Late 2020, diagnosed with cancer to the trigeminal nerve in the right side of the face.
- Lots of very strong med's, at one stage I counted 11, some for pain, others for side effects of meds.

- April 2021, 12 hours of surgery to remove cancer and undergo facial reconstruction. Lymph nodes removed.
- Two days after surgery, my husband was diagnosed with his own blood cancer, not curable but treatable. "It's not a competition", I was heard to say.
- Five days in hospital and back home.

This is where the real journey begins.

- A must have, 'good family and friends as a support network.'
- Know how to accept constructive help and giving clear guidelines on how people can help. Deflect sympathy that has no tangible help.
- Always continue to question and seek answers. Keep trying new solutions and treatments to find what works for you.
- Remember that all specialists that you see are experts in his or her own field but do not have the overall guide to your recovery. Often appointments are 15 minutes, 30 if it's the first consultation or if there is a complication. Take an advocate to important consultations, don't be shy to have a written list of questions and at times I even asked permission to make an audio recording on my phone. Your GP should help you with this journey. This was not possible in my case due to the pandemic and then he left for Australia. He has yet to be replaced in the practice. This is a mine field that you must persist and navigate yourself.
- You are your own advocate in this journey even if you are ill equipped at the outset. It is a very steep learning curve.
- On the 23rd December that year, my dad died on his 85th birthday, the cusp of Christmas. Same cancer, different part of the head. Due to Covid restrictions we had a private family wake. "It was great". A personal send off at my sister's home with good food and wine. Dad's coffin left to "Let's go surfing" by the beach boys belting out down the road. He had been a volunteer lifeguard at wild west coast surf beaches his entire life. This led me to reading the book "With The End In Mind" by Kathryn Mannix. A must read that left me feeling, as a family we had "done good by my dad". I would go so far to say that understanding death, and financial literacy, are skills no longer taught in today's world, at the peril of our youth.

Treatments

- 2021. Surgery, followed 6 weeks later with chemo and radiation. Surgery and chemo were OK. Radiation, not so. Being bolted in a head mask to a table 5 sessions a week for 6 weeks is not fun especially when you know it's not good for the brain. On finishing the treatment my radiologist said "Helen, this is one of the most difficult treatments we offer, you scored a 95% for effort". "No shit Sherlock, I worked that out for myself", I said. "I gave myself a score of 100% for effort".
- Yes, I knew that lymph nodes are tested during cancer surgery, having witnessed my mother's breast cancer journey. With an overload of information to my own situation, it never occurred to me to ask about my own treatment in this area. I was to learn after surgery that 40-50 lymph nodes were removed in the face and neck, all testing negative. "Happy days? No!". The loss of these lymph nodes has caused me problems and moving forward will continue to do so. Please, doctors and surgeons, inform your patients and give them choices. If I had been offered a choice, operate, and test a sample of the lymph nodes, and if the outcome was poor and I had to have a second surgery at my own expense, I would have chosen to do so.
- Not for one moment should people in my post recovery feel that it's OK to treat me by video consultations. They cannot examine me, feel for anomalies or problems or truly understand my pain and fears. I now refuse to see these people via video, as they can only write a script for drugs I can no longer tolerate. My money is better spent elsewhere.

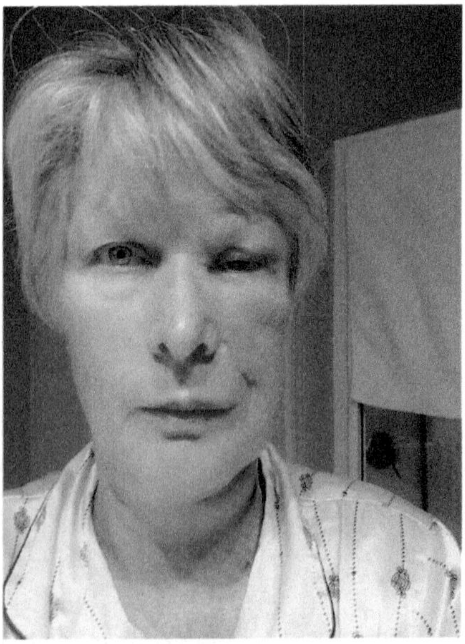

Helen MacLean Pre-Lymphatic Massage - Sept 2022

I have met some truly dedicated and inspiring professionals along the way in my post treatment journey. I continue to have an open mind and am prepared to celebrate any improvement, no matter how small it appears at the time. They all add up to significant change.

These are the post treatments to date which are mainly self-funded with the support of my husband. Hospital and specialist appointments remain a three-way split between National Health, insurance and myself. The more time goes on the greater the self-funding required.

- Jaw specialist. Unable to open my mouth due to shrinkage caused by scarring after radiation. Used a jaw expander, ridiculously expensive but effective.
- Corrective eye lid surgery. Due to no muscle or nerves in the right side of the face causing the lower eye lid to be drooped and tears continually ran down my face. Eye lid had a resection.
- Pain is still ongoing. I'm no longer tolerant of medications. They upset my stomach and bowels.

Solutions

- Meditation. Not for me, I'm too impatient.
- Gratitude. Fantastic, quick, and easy to incorporate into my day. Great attitude changer.
- Specialist head and neck physio. Did internal manipulation in the mouth to open jaw and free up movement in the neck. Lymphatic massage as face very swollen. Also used a Lazer to reduce lymphatic swelling. The skin on the donor site to the arm was stuck to the muscle and bone. A snake bite suction kit was used to pull the skin away creating a gap for the fissure aiding lymphatic and nerve healing. These treatments made a huge difference, and I can now wake up without my eye being seriously swollen.
- Exercise. A little often to bring back normality in daily life and everyday tasks.
- My eyebrows never grew back fully so I now have very subtle tattooed ones.
- Hospital put me on a pain management programme to change attitude to daily pain. Due to Covid this was online. Totally inappropriate for my situation. Head trauma, vision problem, brain fog and an inability to tolerate screen time.
- Became a volunteer on a pain study with Exsurgo. (EEG Neurotherapy Drug Free Chronic Pain Therapy) *https://exsurgo.com* This works by creating new

pathways within the brain, neuroplasticity. Although this didn't work for me, possibly due to age I believe in the science and would not discount it for others. It was a privilege to be included in the programme.

- Lymphatic massage, (2023). Working on creating separation in the fissure between skin, muscle and bone, thus repairing some of the lymphatic and nerve system in the face. It has had pleasing results, reducing swelling and making my face more symmetrical, evening out skin tone and balance. Seldom does my eyelid droop at the end of the day due to tiredness as it had always done before this treatment.
- Almost 2 years on I spend 20 minutes on awaking doing jaw stretchers and lymphatic massage. It works and I will continue to do this for the rest of my life.
- I lost some of my hearing to chemo and a second operation to the ear. Solution, I now use hearing aids.
- I live at the beach but can no longer put my head under the water. With no muscle in the lower eye lid, it acts as a water scoop (bit like a pelican) and is very uncomfortable. Solution, surfer's goggles.
- I'm sensitive to light especially outdoors. Solution, I wear a hat and sunglasses. I drive with the visor down to reduce glare.
- I still enjoy all my outdoor pursuits, although I have to try that little bit harder due to balance and depth perception changes.

Top tip and greatest regret

- Actually, there are two top tips.
- Live each day as it comes. Every day is full of small, but beautiful moments. Sights, sounds and smells; encounters with others and the way you interpret and integrate these moments into our lives; and being comfortable with the new you. The latter being much harder than it sounds.
- Do your lymphatic massage every day, and I mean every day. From time to time, I skip a day or two. My sister with non-Hodgkin's cancer, is quick to remind me. "Helen, you have caught the, 'can't be arsed factor'". This phenomenon developed during the Covid lockdowns. The outcome being, a pudgy, wudgy face. That's enough to motivate me back into action.

- Regrets, just one. The permanent loss of my natural smile with both the mouth and eyes. Yes, my surgeon told me the right side of my face would have no nerve and be paralysed. Reconstructive surgery would use muscle from my arm "which arm would I like to sacrifice?", and that they would implant a gold weight into my eye lid to assist blinking. To be fair, the blink is a little arrested and reminds me of one of those old-fashioned dolls that lay in the bottom of the toy box. When you tipped it up, one eye was always slower to blink than the other. A free and un-arrested smile now looks more like a grimace and has the potential to scare children. "Not always bad, as I work with children and sometimes it works in my favour". But honestly, the fact that I feel the need to arrest every smile in order to look OK, does leave me with a genuine sense of loss. Oh, to smile for a day.

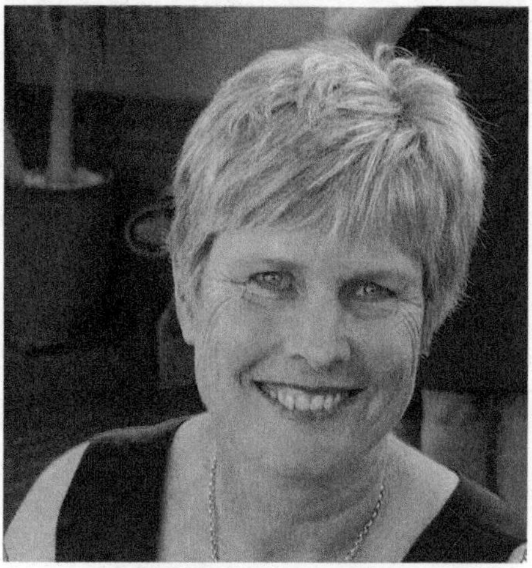

Helen MacLean Pre-Cancer Journey

In January 2023 I celebrated my 60th birthday with family and friends. No mean feat, while in the middle of one of New Zealand most devastating cyclones, there was no way of stopping me! Early February 2023 my surgeon announced me cancer free. I will always be very grateful to my surgeon, Nick, a truly generous and skilled professional and my radiologist, Peppi, who worked tireless hours to map my treatment. Many thanks to all those who have helped me on this journey. Happy days! Not yet pain free but working on it.

TOP TIP!

Live each day as it comes. Every day is full of small, but beautiful moments. Be comfortable with the new you. Remember to do your lymphatic massage every day!

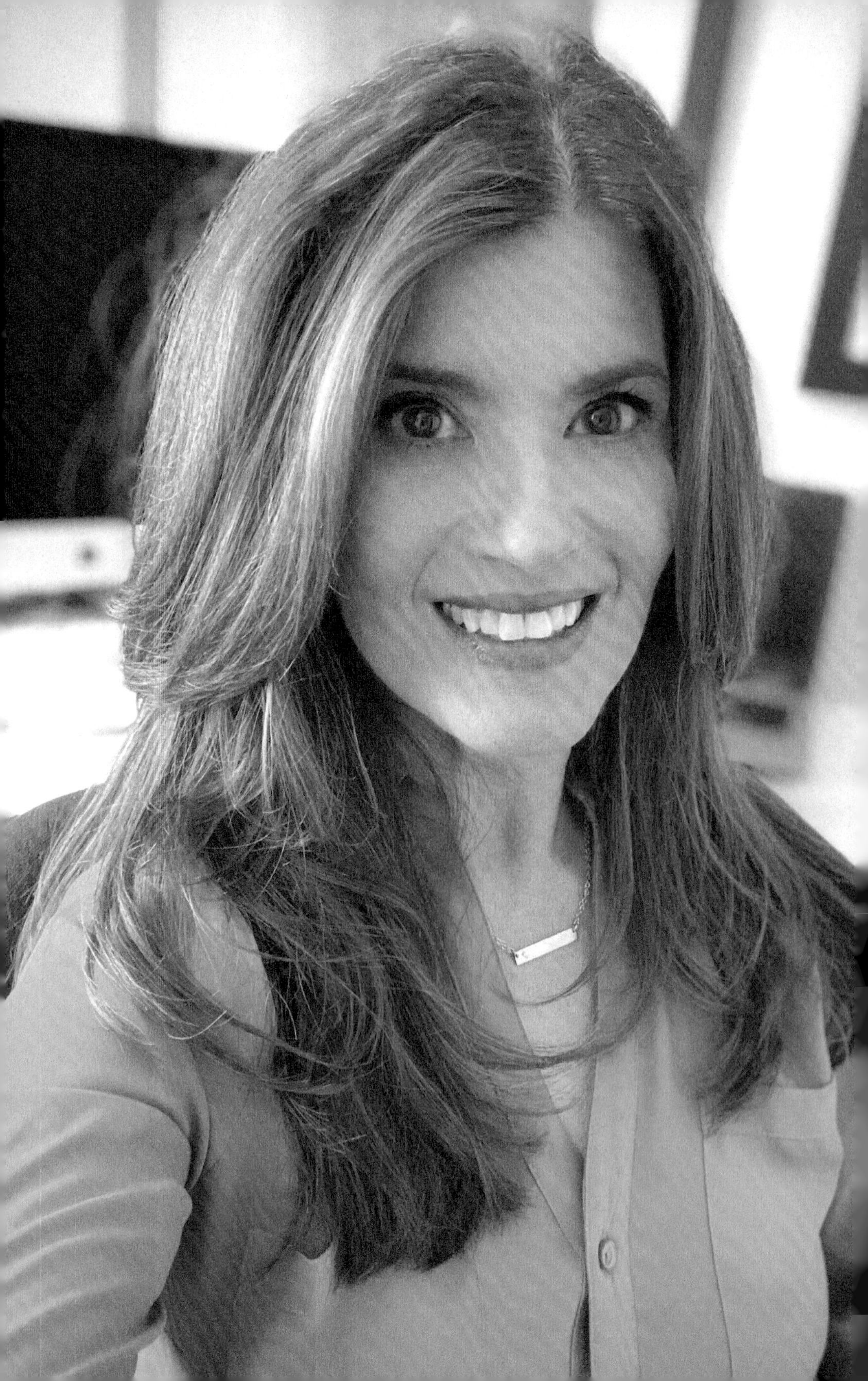

12

ANGELA MARQUEZ

> ***I continued living my life with a new resilience, and I've come through the other side stronger.***

"You have cancer", three words I never expected to hear from my doctor.

In December of 2006, I was diagnosed with cervical cancer and underwent a radical hysterectomy, with the removal of 36 lymph nodes, including an excruciating six weeks of chemotherapy. Next came 35 radiation treatments, followed by four sessions of brachytherapy. That day remains vivid in my mind because the doctor told me that if I was too far gone, he wouldn't operate on me.

I continued living my life with a new resilience, and I've come through the other side stronger.

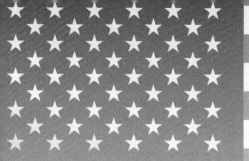

However, in March of 2016, I noticed that my left ankle was swollen. I had tweaked it earlier in the week, so his swelling didn't strike me as unusual. Within a week, and without any apparent cause or provocation, my entire leg swelled up like an inner tube.

My doctor, Dr. Vorhees, asked me to go to the ER, where I was diagnosed with venous insufficiency. With this diagnosis in hand and after going through all of my symptoms and listing possible causes, I knew something wasn't right: *This would end up being my first call for self-advocacy.*

I returned to see my primary doctor, who was not in, and I was seen by another physician. She said, "It's not that bad"; however, when asked if she had a diagnosis for the swollen leg, her response was simply "That's normal." Again, I pushed back against this answer and insisted it be investigated further. I went through visits with various doctors over the course of six weeks asking about the same issue; *"Why is my left foot/leg swelling?".*

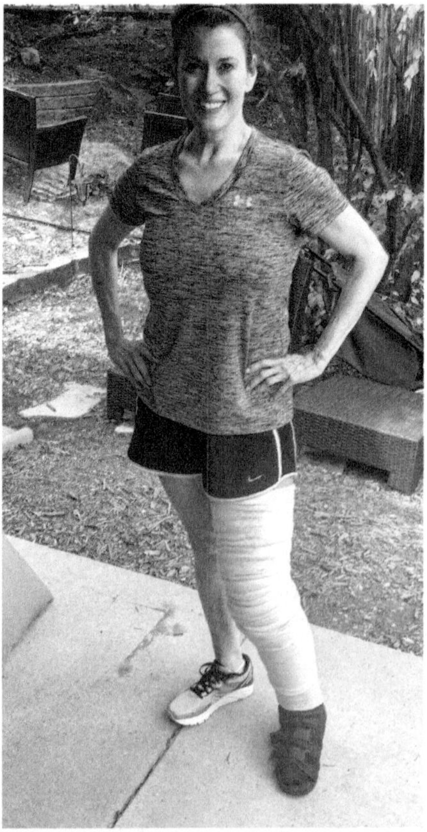

Angela Marquez in wraps

Dr. Vorhees took the time to come in on his day off and spent well over an hour with me. He referred me to an interventional radiologist (IR), who performed a series of tests before determining that I had May Thurner Syndrome (MTS). This occurs when the right iliac artery is compressing the left iliac vein. A stent would need to be inserted because my vein was more than 50% compressed. After a moment of silence, he asked me if I had ever been through any trauma. When I told him that nine years before, I'd been diagnosed with cancer, the expression on his face changed. I could tell he was thinking hard about something.

I was upset and anxious from this news of having MTS and the need for a stent to be placed in my pelvis area. *How would this condition impact my life?* But that's not as upsetting as what I felt when Dr. Rajebi, my Interventional Radiologist, called me to say he thought I also had Lymphedema.

In one week, I was diagnosed with a condition that could be taken care of with stent placement and another disease – lymphedema – without a cure. After my stent was surgically placed, Dr Rajebi asked me to wait an entire month before making a final call on whether he believed I had lymphedema. We wanted to see if the swelling would subside after placement of the stent. My oncologist had mentioned lymphedema as a possible side effect of treatment, and it would usually occur within three years after cancer diagnosis. Since I was more than three years past my initial diagnosis — and closer to nine years — it never occurred to me that I could still develop this disease.

In the time leading up to my appointment with Dr. Rajebi, I immersed myself in information about lymphedema. At that time, there wasn't much available, and what was out there wasn't very promising. It was frustrating to say the least!

I met with Dr. Rajebi a month later and he confirmed I had lymphedema. I had prepared myself for this and hearing the words gave it confirmation. My first question and biggest concern was if I could continue to exercise with lymphedema. This is the one thing I did not want taken away. He said, "Yes, in fact I encourage you to." He said to continue doing all the things I had been doing before my diagnosis. I was relieved and excited to hear this; it brought a bit of normalcy for me. Both Dr. Rajebi and Dr. Voorhees credits self-advocacy and my determination for finding answers, as the basis for me getting diagnosed. Always remember, we are our best advocates!

Shortly after, I was referred to my amazing lymphedema therapist, Vicki Ralph, by Dr. Rajebi (IR doctor). Vicki suggested I bring someone to video me being bandaged. So, I recruited Aaron, my husband, to join me for my appointment; I highly recommend this as we have referred to this video many times. As you can imagine, I was anxious and nervous when I arrived for my appointment. Vicki assured me we would get the swelling down and she really put my mind at ease. I started my Complete Decongestive Therapy (CDT). Vicki gave me manual lymphatic massage treatments three or four times per week while staying bandaged/wrapped for 22 hours except when showering. I continued all my normal activities, working and exercising while in treatment. This helped me mentally as well as physically. Each week I saw progress on the reduction of my leg and that kept me motivated. I kept this routine up for seven weeks and when the bandages came off on August 3rd, my leg volume reduced in size from 36% to 14%! I was so excited! At this time, I got fitted for a compression garment, night garment and ordered a lymphedema pump. Monthly MLD appointments with Vicki continued as usual.

Remember when I mentioned earlier that I had immersed myself in all things lymphedema? Well, after reading about a surgery called Vascular Lymph Node Transfer (VLNT) and learning it could potentially help prevent the progression of my disease if done early enough, in 2017 I decided to have VLNT surgery with Dr. Dayan at Memorial Sloan Kettering Cancer Center in New York City. Although I knew surgery was not a cure, I wanted to do everything in my power to improve the quality of life and slow down the progression of this disease. The surgery has improved my symptoms: I have less tingling and heaviness in my leg, and better mobility as a result. Today, I continually encourage anyone who is considering lymphedema surgery to do their homework and talk with patients, therapists, and surgeons about their experiences. It's not for everyone and it's a decision that should not be taken lightly. These conversations and research can help you make an informed decision, the best decision for you!

Managing this disease is a full-time job, and I am vigilant about my care. However, that doesn't mean I never have flare-ups with my lymphedema. I have had bouts of cellulitis, which at one point kept me in the hospital for a week, leaving me with an intravenous tube inserted in my arm for three weeks. I wear compression garments daily, use a lymphedema pump and night garment, see my CLT and exercise regularly, all to help manage this disease. The standard gold treatment of lymphedema is compression bandaging, manual lymphatic drainage, exercise, diet, and skincare. As for exercise, I find lifting weights helps best manage my lymphedema; I believe the muscle's pumping action helps move the lymph fluid. Exercise is important overall, especially for those of us with lymphedema, no matter how you move; walk, yoga, swim, etc., it all moves the lymph and releases good endorphins!!

I have lived with lymphedema for some time now and I try to live my life to the fullest. When first diagnosed with lymphedema it felt isolating and hard to process. It takes a toll mentally and physically. It is important to reach out to someone you can talk to, and there are lymphedema support groups in person and online. There is no right or wrong way to show up. You are not alone. The same goes for wearing your compression garment; wear it discreetly or for the world to see. Do what feels best for you. For me, wearing my garment to be seen is liberating and if someone asks, it gives me the opportunity to educate them about lymphedema.

I want to thank my family and friends who have helped and supported me. Aaron—my best friend and husband—for all that you have done and continue to do and for learning to wrap; so that you could bandage me. Throughout this

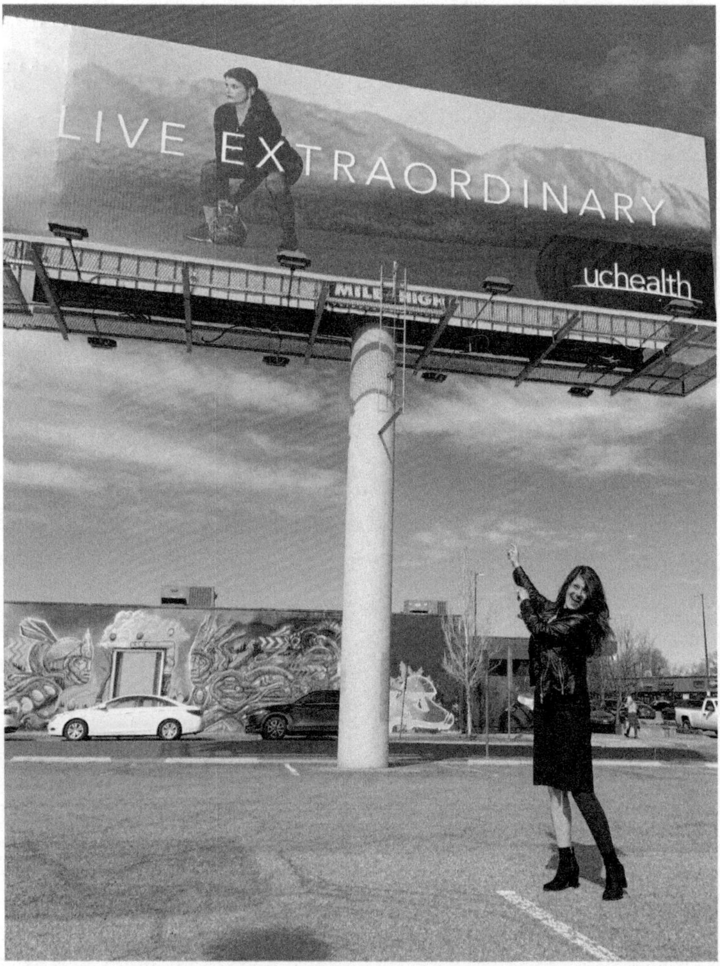

Angela Marquez - Poster Billboard - Pointing in the right direction!

journey, my gracious family has supported me and my cause. My friends have been there for me throughout. I am forever grateful!

I use my voice to bring awareness to this disease. I volunteer for the Lymphatic Education & Research Network (LE&RN), a non-profit organization whose mission is to fight lymphatic disease through education, research, and advocacy. As a volunteer I speak to various groups about lymphedema; meet with lymphedema support groups; organize fundraisers and serve on the advisory board for the University of Colorado Hospital—a Center of Excellence (COE). The COE designation is given to healthcare organizations that provide comprehensive services and care for patients with Lymphatic Diseases (LD).

I have an Instagram account (@funky_lymphedema) where I share awareness, living life with lymphedema, connect with others, and hope to motivate others with this disease to live their life to the fullest, not allowing it to be a barrier. I created the Instagram account because when I was researching lymphedema, I quickly realized there was a need for awareness and positive-motivating information about this disease. Most of what I found was not presented in this way and it tended to focus on the more negative aspects, rather than people's successes with managing their lymphedema. I have met some remarkable people! The lymphedema community is welcoming, and you'll find support both online and in person. My perseverance through all of this has made me strong and the person I am today!

I want to emphasize that you should always be your own best advocate. No one knows the inner workings of your body better than yourself, so it's crucial that we all stand up for ourselves and raise awareness about this disease! Remember, you are not alone.

I try to keep a positive outlook on things and believe that the mind is an extremely powerful tool. I hope my story helps others, no matter how small or large — if it helps just one person, then it's all worth it!

TOP TIP!

Live your life to the fullest, and don't allow lymphedema or any other condition to be a barrier. Don't give up — ever!

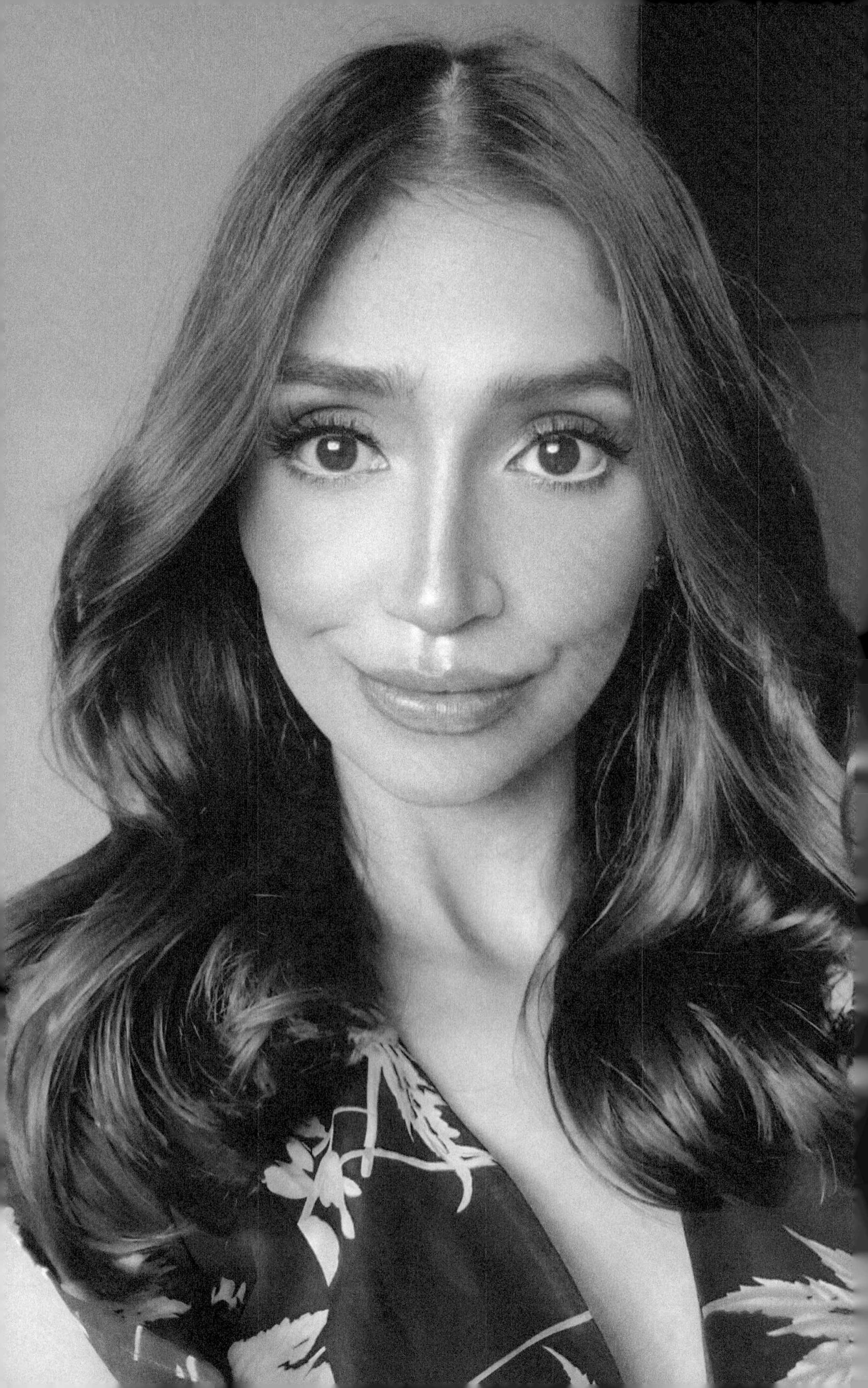

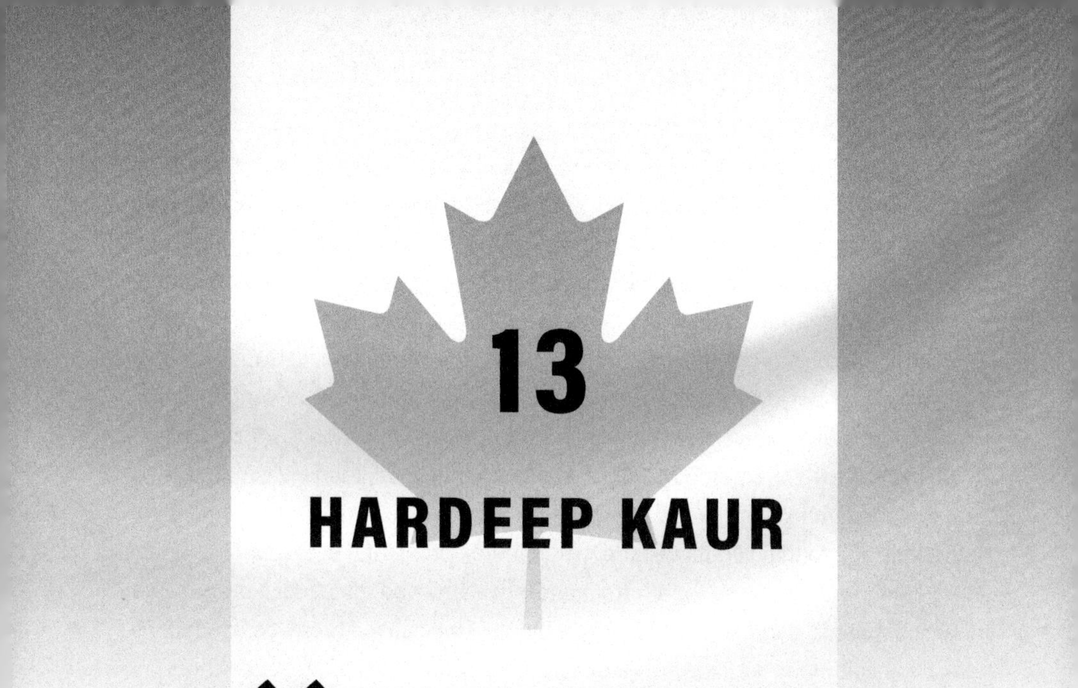

13

HARDEEP KAUR

> ***This was another defining moment in my life. I was a teenager who went through a near-death experience.***

My story begins in Toronto, Canada on October 1st, 1987, at Humber River Hospital. I was 6.5 lbs and I was placed in an incubator for a few weeks because I was not doing well. My mom was also not doing well. After my health stabilized my mom and I were discharged from the hospital. Everything seemed fine for a while after that, until the 6-month mark. My parents noticed the Indian bangles on my right wrist were starting to get tighter and tighter because my hand and arm were starting to swell. My parents didn't understand what was happening. I was their firstborn, and they were new immigrants to Canada at the time who didn't speak or understand English fluently, so I can only imagine the stress they felt. They proceeded to take me to the family doctor. The family doctor wasn't sure what was happening, and he referred me to Sick Kids Hospital in downtown Toronto. My parents almost immediately took me there and pretty quickly I was diagnosed with primary lymphedema in my right arm and hand. I know I was one of the lucky ones who got diagnosed very quickly.

Now that I had a diagnosis my parents and I had to learn how to live with this condition. What was lymphedema? We had to learn as much as we could because we didn't know anyone else with this condition. I was very young when I was diagnosed so I don't remember much, but my parents and grandparents did everything they could while working full-time jobs to take care of me. I often think about the struggles my parents faced, as new immigrants to Canada, with a newborn, who had a rare disease. Sick Kids Hospital was not near our house and my parents didn't have a car back then so they would take public transportation to take me to my numerous doctors' appointments. Back then I wasn't provided a lymphedema pump to use at home, my mom would take me to the hospital periodically so that I could use the lymphedema pump at the hospital. I not only had lymphedema in my right arm/hand but I also had intestinal lymphedema which meant I had gastrointestinal problems. This caused many complications in my health journey. I was on a special diet from an early age, even though I didn't always follow it. I just wanted to be a kid. I wanted to be carefree. I wanted to be like everyone else. One fond memory I have is something that probably sounds so silly, but I was not allowed to drink 2% milk because I couldn't digest it. I would have to drink this nasty formula that smelled horrific, but it was loaded with nutrients that I was able to digest. But I wanted to drink 2% milk! So, I would go to the fridge and sneakily drink some 2% milk hoping my parents wouldn't catch me and they never did haha (at least that's what I think). I had so many restrictions on what I could and could not eat/drink from an early age.

The years went on and I tried to live a normal life. I started going to school. Being the first child of immigrant parents meant English was my second language and Punjabi my first. No one at home spoke English at that point. So aside from having the normal first-generation Canadian life struggles, I also had to overcome the struggles of being a kid with lymphedema. Sometimes kids at school were mean because they didn't understand what was wrong with my arm and hand. I also didn't have the vocabulary to explain what happened to my arm and hand, because I myself didn't understand why my hand and arm were swollen and big. I remember wearing a beige-colored compression garment every day. That was the only color available back then but that was fine by me because I just wanted to blend in with everyone else. I remember one day at recess in grade 2 or 3, I was playing with a girl and she went to reach for my right hand and stopped after she noticed I had a glove on my hand. That was a defining moment in my life. I think that was one of the first times I started feeling weird, ugly, and different.

While struggling with living with lymphedema I was also struggling with my overall health. I was hospitalized many times over the years for extended amounts of time because my body was not absorbing nutrients from the food and supplements I was eating. I was extremely deficient in so many vitamins and minerals, this condition is called malabsorption which is a side effect of my intestinal lymphedema. When I was 10 years old I had to learn how to put a feeding tube through my nose because the food I was eating was not being digested properly and I also wasn't growing in terms of my height. Doctors decided the feeding tube might help me get the nutrients I needed and might help me grow. Every night I would put a feeding tube in my nose, and through the feeding tube, I would administer a formula that ran through it all night. I remember it smelled horrible. Alongside this I still had to take supplements, to give you a better understanding of how deficient I was. Here's an example, I had to take 27 vitamin E pills a day! I would take 9 three times a day, this was just vitamin E, not all the other pills I took. At that time my lymphedema took a backseat. I was just struggling to survive.

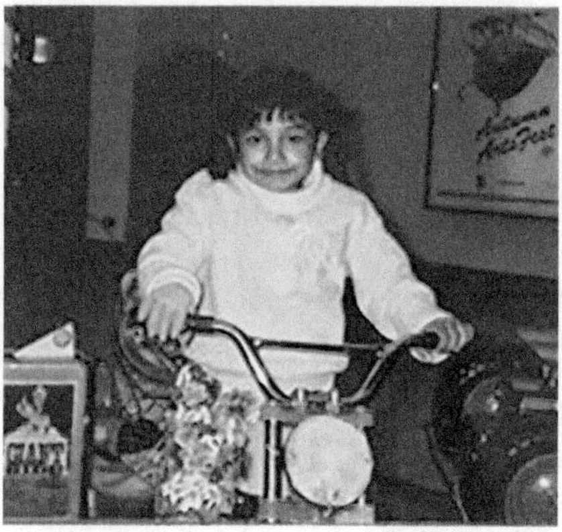

Hardeep Kaur – I just wanted to be a kid!

When I was 15, I became extremely ill. I was hospitalized for malnutrition, then it got worse, I suffered a cardiac arrest and kidney failure during my hospitalization. I was put into an induced coma while the doctors tried to stabilize my health. It was a scary time. I don't remember all of it. I remember bits and pieces. I remember thinking I was going to die. I knew it didn't look good for me. I wasn't able to breathe on my own, and all my organs were failing. The doctors told my parents I was the sickest kid in Sick Kids Hospital at that time and that they didn't think I'd make it. Not something any parent wants to hear. Somehow, I beat the odds and recovered. I had to learn how to walk again because I had been in a hospital bed for such a long time. I had to learn how to inject myself with blood thinners in my thigh. I lost almost all my hair. After spending 5 months in the hospital, I was finally discharged. This was another defining moment in my life. I was a teenager who went through a near-death experience.

I went back to high school after I was discharged from the hospital. I hated high school. For one I was bullied, I felt like an outcast, a loner. People in high school would refer to me as the girl with the big arm. I never fit in because I wasn't like any of the kids I knew. How many teenagers do you know that have a rare disease like lymphedema and go through a near-death experience by the age of 15. Probably not that many! I wasn't relatable. I didn't know it then but looking back now I know I was depressed during that time. I graduated high school a few years late and went on to university not having a clue what I was doing or who I was. I still didn't know what lymphedema really was, how I got it, or anyone else who had it. I kept hiding it like I always had, going far as wearing jackets in the summer just so people wouldn't see my arm. I would feel so hot and uncomfortable, but I didn't care, I didn't want anyone to see my arm. I still wasn't taking care of my lymphie arm properly, I didn't wear my compression garment regularly, I never pumped, and I never bandaged my arm. My arm was very big at this point. My self-esteem was very low. I just wanted to disappear.

Life went on. I graduated from university and went on to do a post-graduate program. By then I was in my late twenties. I started working on my self-esteem, learning who I was, and trying to navigate life at the same time. I remember on the first day that I started my post-graduate program we all had to introduce ourselves by saying our name, and one thing about us to the class. I decided to tell the class my arm is swollen because I have lymphedema. That was a big step for me. I did that because I knew I would inevitably get questions about it, so I wanted to get ahead of that and just put it out there. Slowly but surely small steps like that built my confidence.

During my twenties, I started watching YouTube videos and started learning how to apply makeup. It slowly became one of my passions. To this day I love applying makeup and learning makeup techniques and I love how it can transform how you feel and look. People started complimenting my makeup skills and saying I was pretty. Being called pretty felt so foreign to me. I never thought I was pretty. It did something for my confidence. I started believing I was pretty. Makeup made me feel like I had an alter ego, finally, the attention was on something other than my arm. Makeup became my escape. As I've gotten older and now that I'm in my mid-30s I still love makeup and the power of makeup, but I don't need it to feel beautiful anymore. I don't use makeup to distract people from my lymphie arm anymore.

I've done so much work on myself and there's always more work to do, but I feel more confident in my skin than I ever have. I wear tank tops, short sleeve shirts, and bright-colored compression garments. Most importantly now, I take care of my lymphedema. I do everything in my power every day to keep the swelling down because I understand self-care and consistency are everything when it comes to managing this lifelong condition. As for my overall health, I still struggle with other health problems aside from lymphedema and sometimes it all feels like too much. I still suffer from malabsorption for which I take many supplements every day, I get ultrasounds of my kidneys regularly because of my history of kidney failure. I recently got diagnosed with thoracic outlet syndrome. Despite all this even when it gets hard, I never give up.

My number one tip for living with lymphedema and thriving is to take care of yourself. For me, that doesn't just mean taking bubble baths and going on vacations. It means eating well, drinking enough water, moving my body, doing things that make me happy, surrounding myself with people who genuinely care about me, and a community of lymphie friends (this one has been life-changing). Sometimes I think back to how lonely I felt before I found so many people with lymphedema. It all started one late night when I was 32 laying in bed, I thought to myself what if I searched the hashtag lymphedema on Instagram? So, I did just that. To my amazement, I found people with lymphedema! I cried tears of joy because I couldn't believe it. I finally saw someone whose arm was swollen like mine. I messaged her right away. From that point forward I kept meeting more and more lymphies online and then in person in Toronto! It's funny

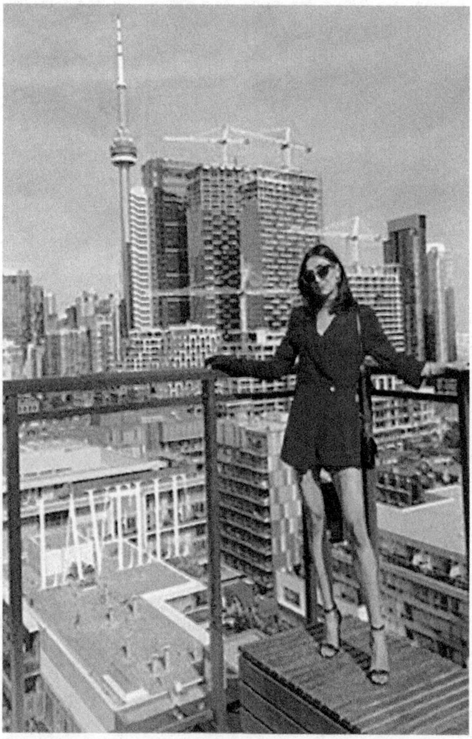

Hardeep Kaur – Thriving with lymphoedema

how life works. I never thought I'd be understood and seen but now I am. I don't ever take it for granted.

The most important thing to remember is you're not alone.

"What you seek is seeking you"

—RUMI

TOP TIP!

Take care of yourself. Eat well, drinking enough water, move your body, do things that make you happy, and surround yourself with people who genuinely care about you, including a community of lymphie friends.

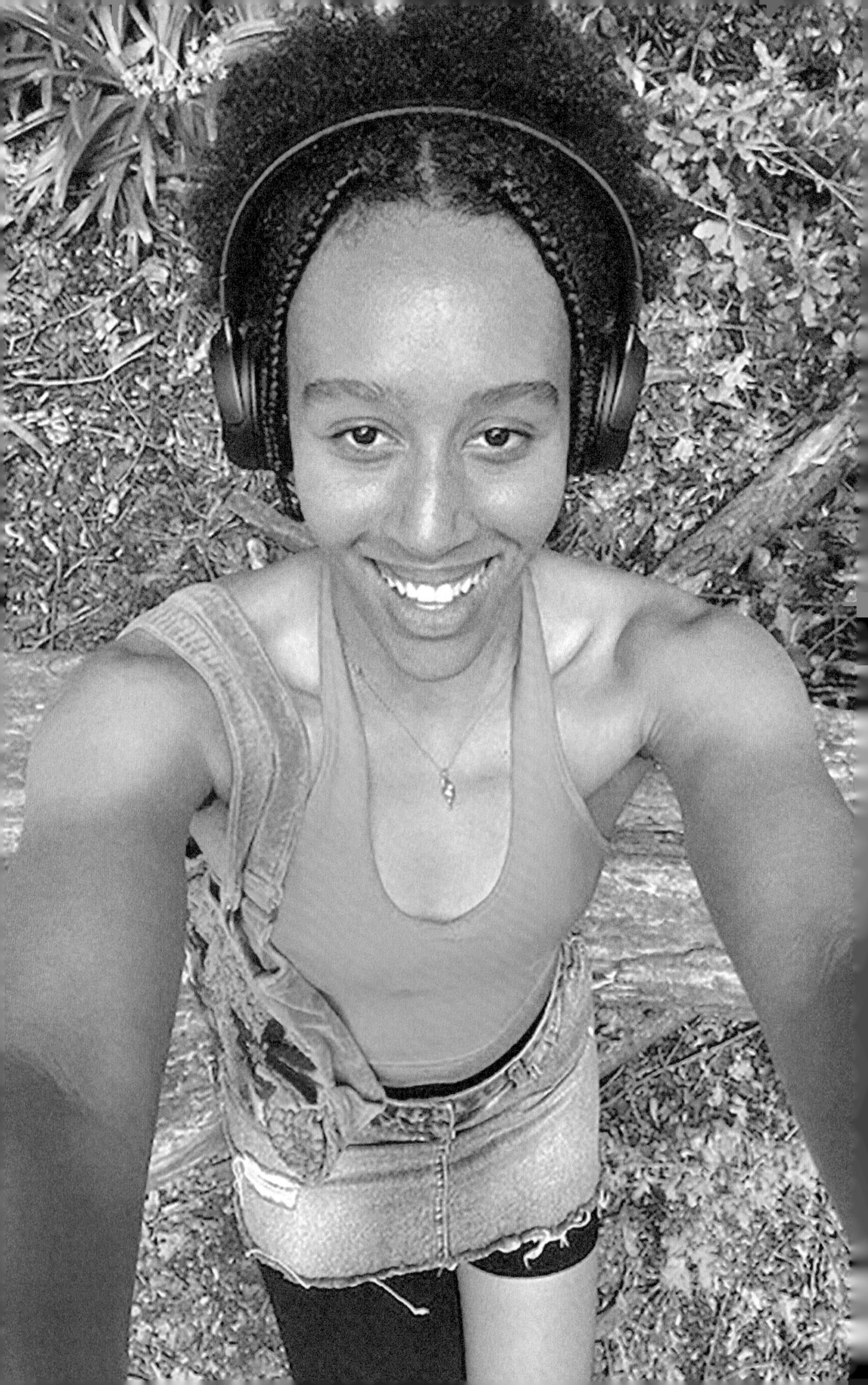

14

DIDI OKOH

> ***I hope that anything I do, no matter how small, will help someone else who's struggling.***

My story starts when I was 12 years old, and I realised my left leg was bigger than the other. It then took 4 years and 3 bouts of cellulitis to be properly diagnosed with primary lymphedema, at the age of 16. I'm now 20 years old and here to share my experiences, and to help others on similar journeys! I hope that anything I do, no matter how small, will help someone else who's struggling.

Before noticing that there was an issue with my leg, I was a very active person and having participated in athletics at a national level, I was aspiring to be a world-class athlete. I had spent my whole childhood partaking in all kinds of sports like ballet, netball, hockey and of course, athletics. But that all rapidly changed one seemingly normal afternoon.

I was 12 years old, taking part in a gifted and talented athletics session when one of my peers mentioned that my left thigh was bigger than the other. At the time, it was hardly noticeable, and we assumed it was my other leg that was the issue because my left leg is my dominant leg within sports (meaning that maybe it was just more muscular). We joked about it, and I carried on with my day. I briefly mentioned it to my parents and coaches, who thought we needed to strengthen my right leg to correct the muscle imbalance. However, nearly a year later I became very ill after doing a cross country race and a netball tournament on the same day. My left leg had come up in red rashes and I was feverish. We would later find out that I actually had cellulitis.

My parents and I then decided to get my leg checked out as it had started to get worse. I continued athletics but put a hold on netball and hockey to lessen the workload on my leg, while we attempted to figure out what was wrong. It was an exhausting process to be suddenly lumped with, at 13 years old, going from one consultant to the other, with one telling me to 'just take Calpol and the swelling will go down.' I have always been a bubbly positive individual, but I really did begin to see the cracks forming in myself. I finally got referred to GOSH (Great Ormond Street Hospital). They ran lots of tests, including a biopsy, and determined I had a lymphatic malformation, but didn't specify what was the problem, or how this came about. The amount of time I spent being investigated through the hospital was enough to make me realise that there was a bigger issue than we had previously thought. However, I didn't let that stop my athletics as I carried on training through this issue and was still performing well at a national level. I can honestly say athletics has always been my safety net and it really helped me stay as upbeat and active as possible. However, from 13-16 years old, my leg gradually deteriorated, with the whole of my left leg from groin to foot starting to become noticeably bigger than the other. At first, I would only feel a very mild pain when exercising, but the pain has progressed rapidly over the years, whereby every day, 24/7, I feel some form of pain ranging from a numbing feeling to a feeling of lactic acid 10times over. This can often prevent me from finishing my training sessions and even from getting out of bed. At 14 years old, I had 3 cellulitis infections in one year. Cellulitis is caused by the slightest of cuts or bites. When I had my first serious cellulitis infection, I was in immense pain, pain that I'd never felt before. I was completely out of it, my mind spinning until everything went black. I never remember too much when I have an infection, just that I am not with it and I can't walk. When I had my first big infection, I became overwhelmed with emotions because I finally understood that my life will never go back to the way it used to be.

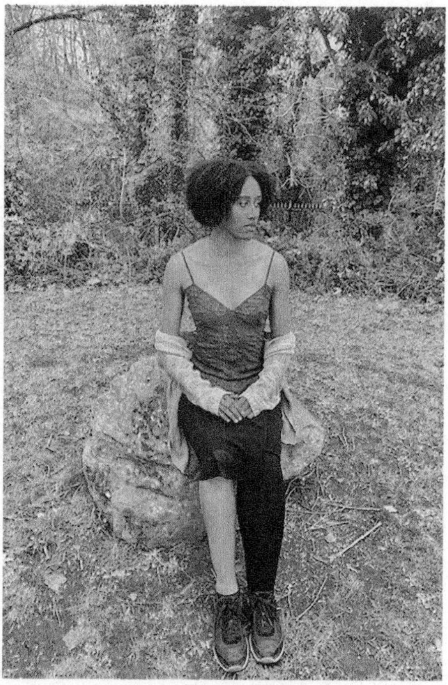

Didi Okoh – Finding her rock

When I turned 16, I was transferred to St. Georges Hospital in London, where I was put under even more tests, including a lymphoscintigram to fully identify the problem. Professor Mortimer then diagnosed me with primary lymphoedema.

During this period of uncertainty, I had at least 3 bouts of cellulitis, which caused my leg to swell and progress further. It got to a point where my doctors put me on prophylactic antibiotics for 3 years (15-18). I'm now 20, as I write this, and still on this course for another 2 years. This is because despite being on the antibiotics, I have had a further 2 infections, making this a total of 5 infections. Having this many infections at such a young age did make me feel helpless, like I was going down a spiral that I could never crawl back up. I was depleted, and I cut off communication with many friends; I was officially isolated from the world.

When I was officially diagnosed, I had many feelings, most of them being negative because I was hitting my prime teenager years and was beginning to feel self-conscious about the size of my leg. I was getting a lot of comments from my school peers, and strangers would stop me on the street to ask what was wrong or would even take pictures of me minding my own business. I had no one to talk to, to relate to, and due to my health, I was so far behind in my education that my teachers wanted me to move down a year. My peers would say I was faking my health problems for attention, which particularly hurt to hear because I just wanted to get through the school year peacefully, I didn't want to be in pain. I had to work extremely hard to pass my GCSE's and take my A-levels, and I've ended up at a Russel group university!

It took a lot of courage and self-development to get myself back on the right path, and I honestly didn't think I was strong enough mentally to deal with such a vigorous condition. There have been too many times to count where I have given up on myself. My lowest moment must have been when I got chucked out of my athletics group because of having lymphedema. They didn't want to coach me because my leg made me an 'injury risk.' That's when I completely shut down. I stopped training, and I stopped caring. My leg size increased drastically which is why the pain has progressed throughout the years. But one day, I came to the realisation that I shouldn't hide away from who I am, and I shouldn't let other people's opinions dictate what I do with my life! The fact that I used to feel so alone is partly why in 2020 I started gradually posting about lymphedema and spreading awareness, so no one should ever have to feel that alone. I want as many people as possible to have the confidence to embrace who they are, without feeling embarrassed or ashamed, particularly those in the younger generations. I know I would've wanted to see someone my age proving to the world that they can do anything anyone else can! I want to be that bubbly, positive person for everyone, and show that having lymphedema isn't going to prevent you from living your life to the fullest.

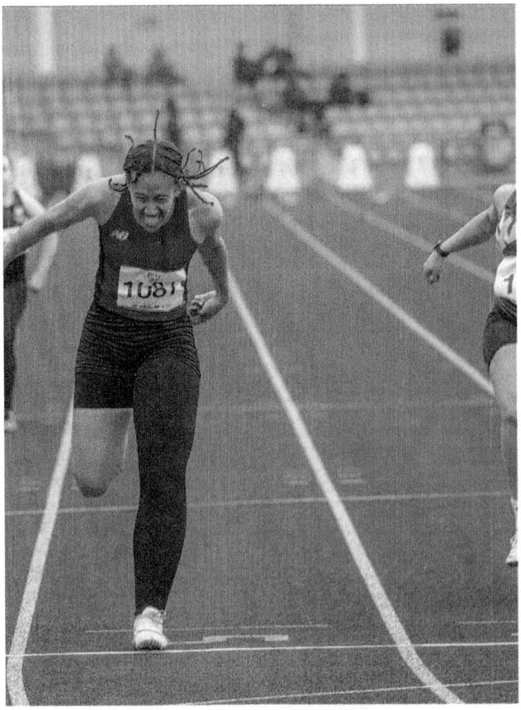
Didi Okoh - Winning her race!

In terms of athletics, I have just been classified as a T44 athlete. I met a lovely individual in my category that made me see that having lymphedema didn't mean I should stop doing what I love to do, just that there was a different path set for me. This is my first season as a para-athlete, and I have already unofficially beaten the European record for long jump in my category! My aims and ambitions, as always, are high for my athletic dreams, and I know I will achieve them. I have also very recently been signed with a modelling agency which I am hoping will allow people living with lymphedema to see themselves in a more positive light through fashion!

Hopefully, I've given a proper insight into what living with lymphedema was like for me as a teenager, and that your journey is still as bright as ever with this condition.

Feel free to follow my Instagram page @didi_okoh and my TikTok page @ didilonglegss as I spread awareness of lymphedema there!

TOP TIP!

Perseverance is so important. Despite the fact you may start to feel your health going 2 steps forward and 1 step back, hold onto things that make you happy, keep at the treatment, and keep smiling!

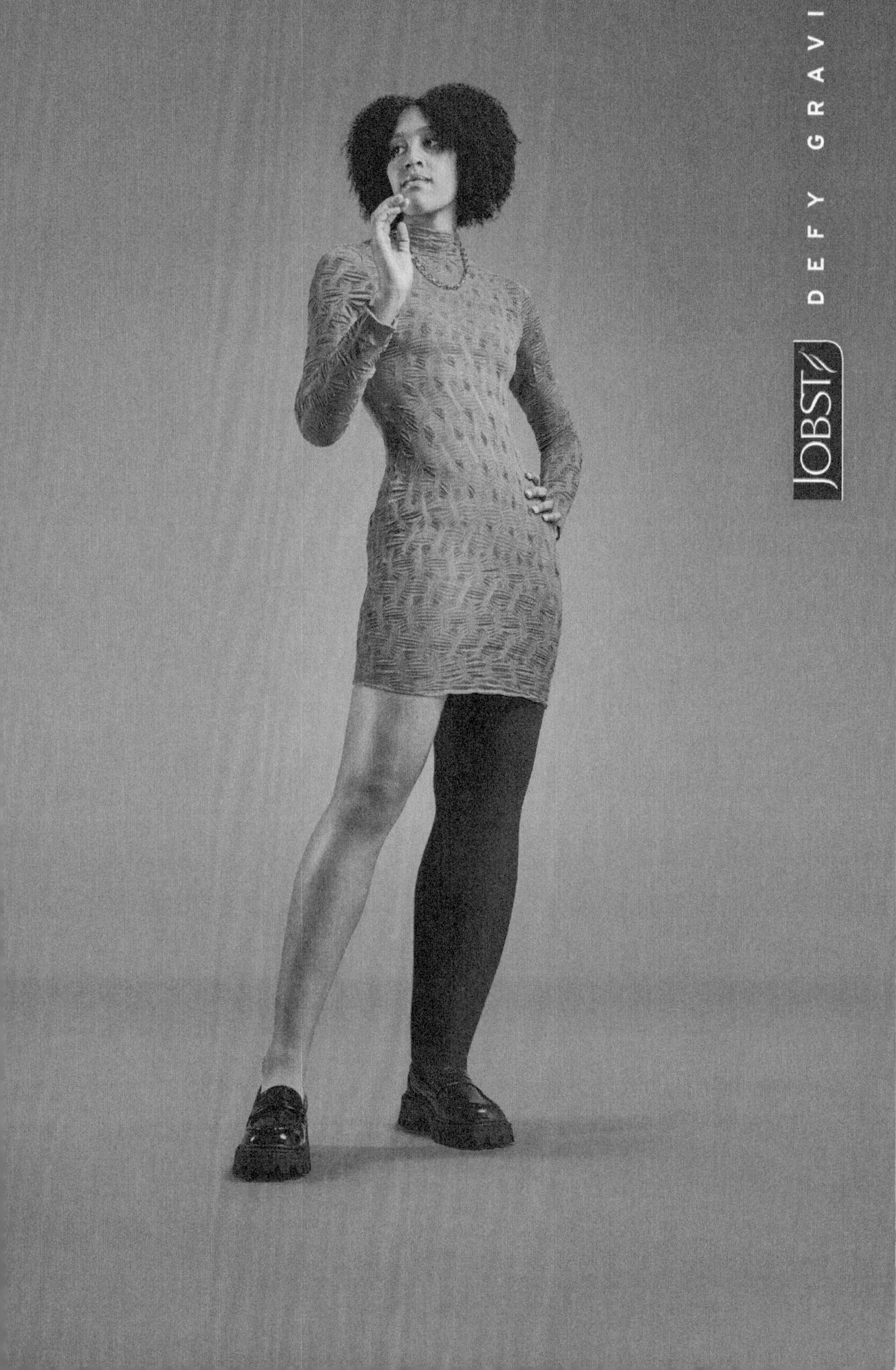
DEFY GRAVITY
JOBST

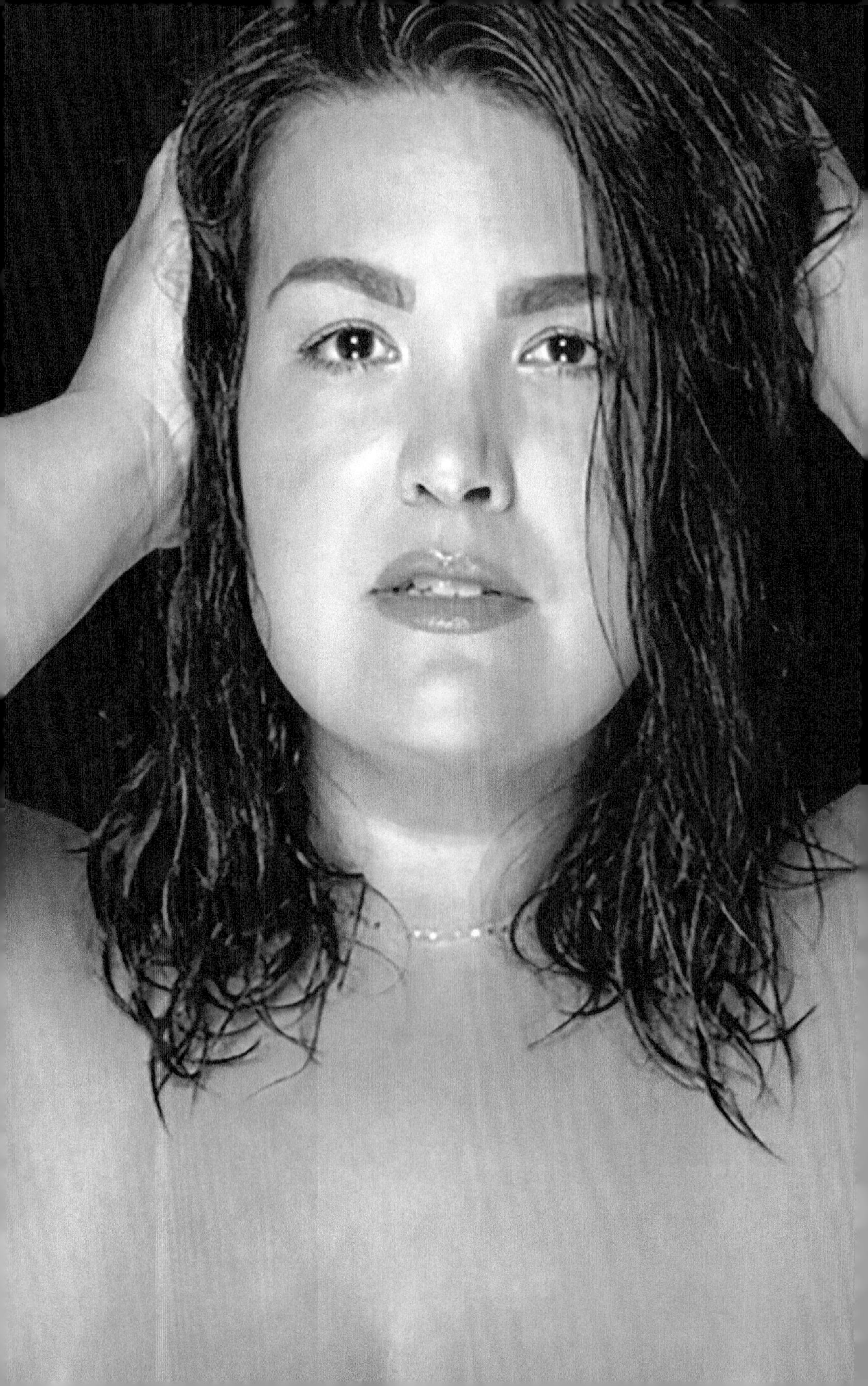

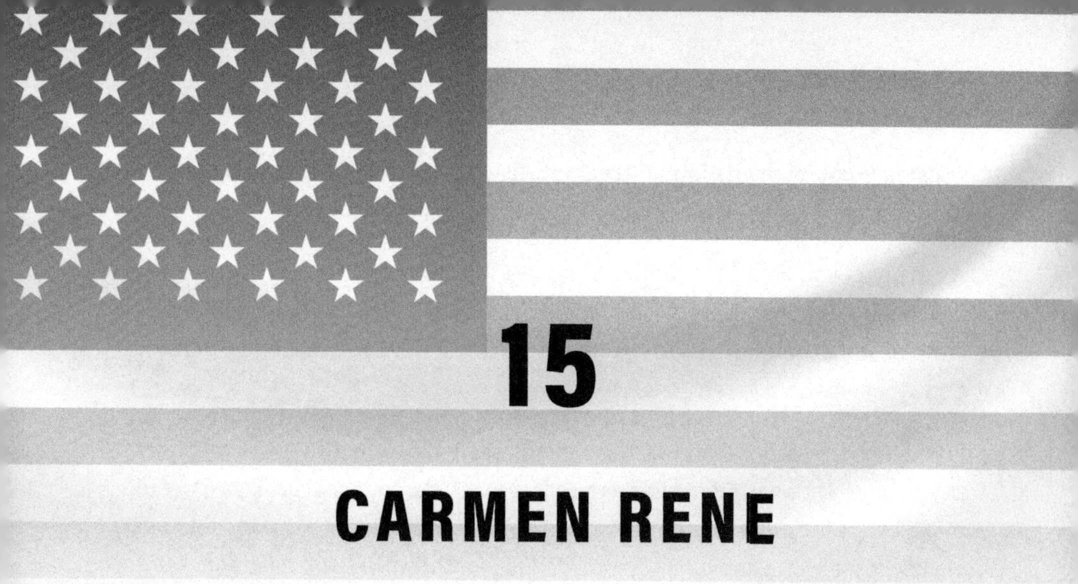

15

CARMEN RENE

> ***It took me a long time to find any type of comfort or confidence with my body, that was so different in so many ways.***

We all have something that makes us different. What we aren't always taught is that those differences are what set us up on the path to stand out and create the change needed in this world.

Growing up as one of the only plus-size kids in my small town came with its challenges as many can relate to. Add swollen legs and feet to the equation and it became a much more lonely journey to navigate. Little did I know, my legs would one day become my superpower to share with the world.

By the age of 3, my mother took me to the doctor with concerns for my feet. I would limp down the stairs every morning and complain that I was in pain. After several appointments and doctors, it was determined that I was likely missing some of my lymph nodes and was given my lymphedema diagnosis at that time.

As many of you know, the diagnosis is only the first step in a very challenging lifelong journey. It took me a long time to know what management tools would work best for me and also to find any type of comfort or confidence with my body that was so different in so many ways.

I remember my Mom trying to make things seem as normal as possible for me by convincing department stores to sell us two different shoe sizes as a set to make up for the extra size on my right side. She controlled what she could but we know the world can be a very cruel place for those who are different.

My body, legs, and feet convinced me that I was somehow unworthy of being loved or experiencing all the joys and adventures life has to offer. Finding out just how untrue that was is where my real story begins.

By my early twenties I started to reassess the relationship I have with my body as a whole and started to decide that hating what I saw in the mirror wasn't working, so why not try loving it instead? By 27, the concept of my social media page started to come together.

Eat The Cake Too was something I developed from that pesky saying "You can't have your cake and eat it too." I always felt that in terms of my body. As if society had already put me in a box of what I can and cannot do, have, wear, or experience based on my size and condition. The mission behind my page has always been to experience life and all it has to offer exactly as you want to and deserve to. No restrictions because of the insecurities of society make us feel. No memories are missed because of the fear of other people's opinions.

A huge part of my social media mission is to continue to spread awareness for both lymphedema and lipedema. Two conditions that often go undiagnosed or misdiagnosed. It has been such an amazing experience to have found and continue to connect with people in our community. I think it is such an important part of social media that often gets overlooked by the negativity a lot of different bodies experience.

When I started sharing my legs and diagnosis, I knew I would receive a lot of negativity but decided it would be worth it to positively impact others with similar stories. I'm happy to say that any trolls are heavily outnumbered by all of the support I receive as well as the women who share how they have started to feel more comfortable in their bodies. That is what I mean when I say our differences are our superpowers! We are changing people's perceptions of chronic illnesses, helping people along their body love journey, and breaking generational cycles! If that isn't a superpower, I don't know what is.

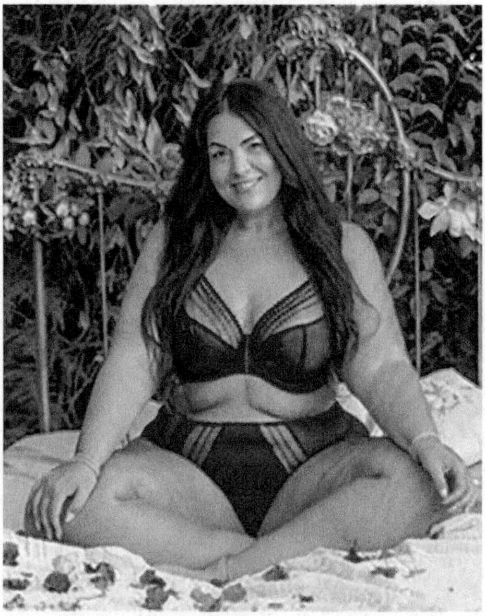

Carmen Rene - My legs are my Superpower!

We have so much life to live and joy to experience despite any challenges lymphedema may bring our way. My advice to anyone struggling is to know that a community is out here waiting to welcome you and you are more powerful and worthy than you give yourself credit for.

TOP TIP!

Keep your head held high, those beautiful lymphie legs elevated, and remember that life is short so you better eat the cake too!

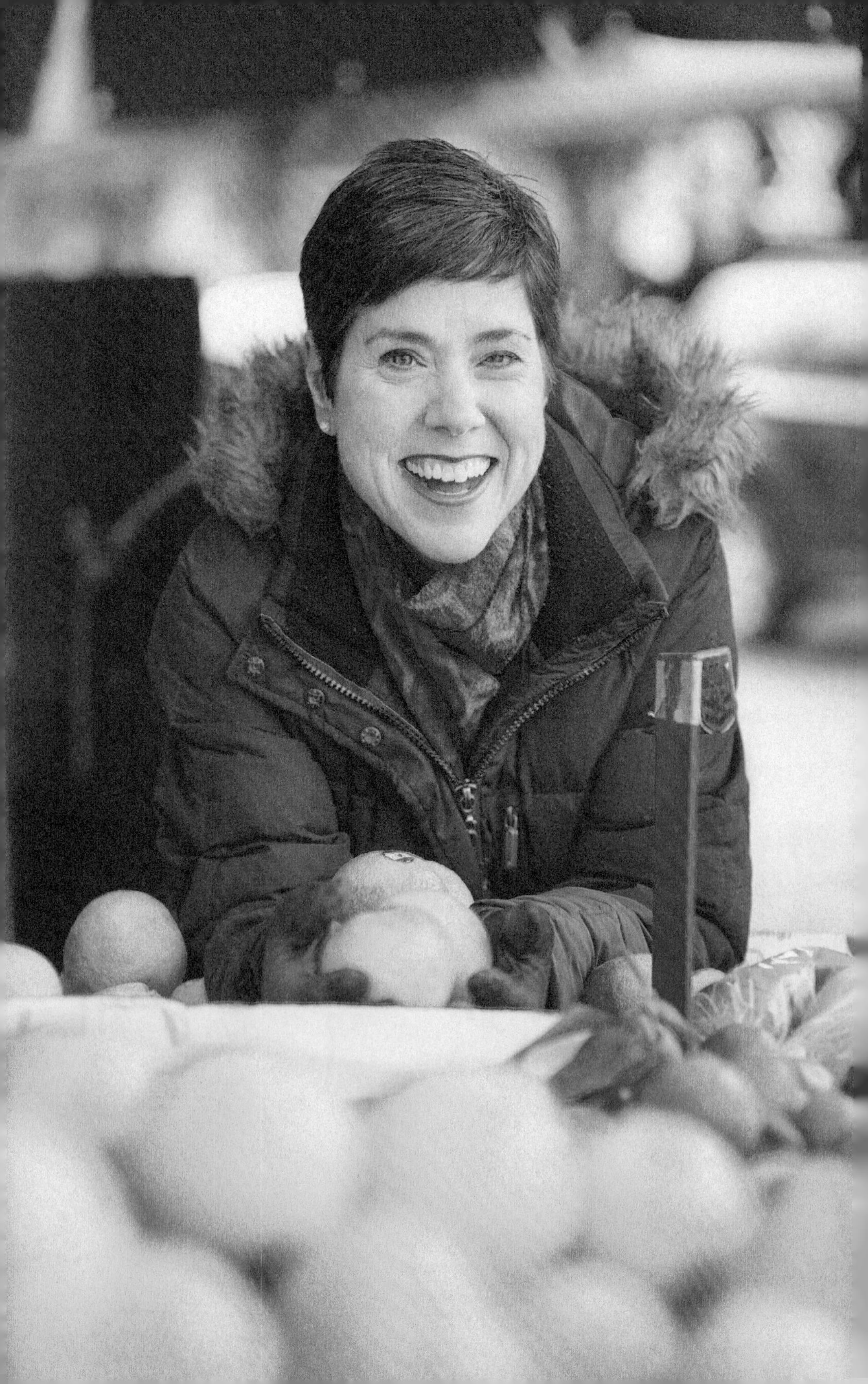

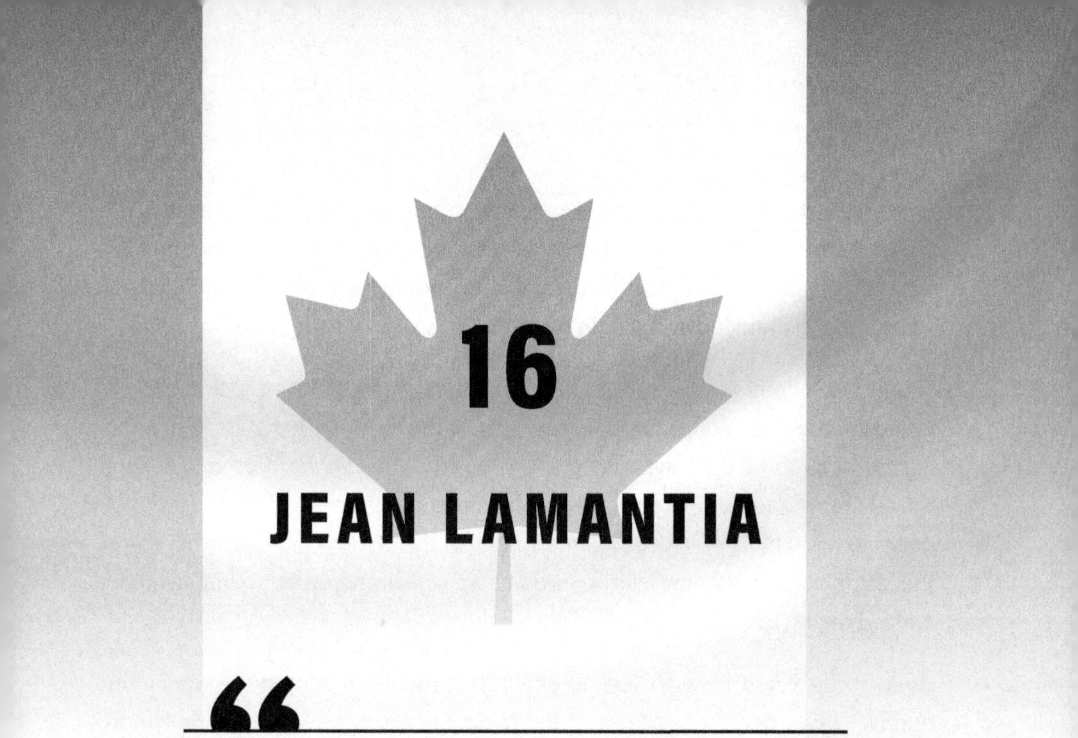

16

JEAN LAMANTIA

> ***Because of the massive and fast-growing tumor in the middle of my chest, that lymphatic fluid was not going into my blood stream, it was being dumped into my lungs.***

I'm a registered dietitian, speaker, author and survivor of lymphoma. Through my experiences I've learned that the lymphatic system is not something trivial to be glossed over in university curriculums, but a vital, highly organized system that responds to touch, compression, diet and more. I'm proud to lead the charge of dietitians to shine a light on the importance of nutrition therapy for lymphedema.

When I was 27 years old, I was diagnosed with Hodgkin's lymphoma – cancer of the lymphatic system. In my case, the lymph nodes in my neck, under both arms and in the middle of my chest were affected. While I can trace my symptoms back seven months prior to my actual diagnosis, despite seeing two different doctors, my cancer was not diagnosed when the symptoms first appeared.

As it turns out, one afternoon, while out of town, I found myself in a shopping mall that had a blood donor clinic. I had previously given blood on four occasions, so I thought, I would go ahead and get my card stamped one more time. But the morning after this donation, I was feeling poorly. My throat started to feel scratchy, and I noticed swelling in my neck.

I knew I was coming down with something and I raced to drive the three hours to my parents' home after dropping a friend at the airport, so that I could nurse myself back to health. The next day, on Good Friday, in addition to the sore throat and tender lymph nodes, I felt a distinctive heaviness in the middle of my chest. My mother instructed me to get to the walk-in clinic. At the clinic, the doctor diagnosed me with bronchitis and gave me an antibiotic, which I started taking.

By Monday, when I wasn't feeling any better, my mom sent me to my family doctor. I described the pressure in the middle of my chest, the swollen lymph nodes in my neck and the peculiar sensation that when I squeezed my arms in at my sides, I could feel bumps in my armpits. My doctor ordered a chest x-ray and sent me on my way.

My family doctor had never called me at home before. But he called and said, I needed to see a doctor right away, but since he was going out of town, he asked me to see his colleague, a respirologist. This was worrisome...my mother (a retired nurse) immediately started going through her rolodex of diseases and wondered...did I have tuberculosis? I had just gotten back from a three-month backpacking trip in Mexico, Belize, Guatemala and Honduras and had been through some very impoverished communities. What else could it be?

We went to the respirologist who immediately started asking about family history of cancer. Suspicions were mounting...then he announced that I had one of two conditions...both of which were cancer. More tests would be needed. My mother and I were in shock. The only thing she managed to get out was "Mario Lemieux". "Yes, the doctor said, Mario Lemieux".

You see, we're Canadian and Mario Lemieux "the magnificent one" is a famous (to Canadians) hockey player (translation: ice hockey player) that was diagnosed with Hodgkin's lymphoma and beat it...and was able to return to hockey. This was the kind of positive example that the doctor wanted us to focus on.

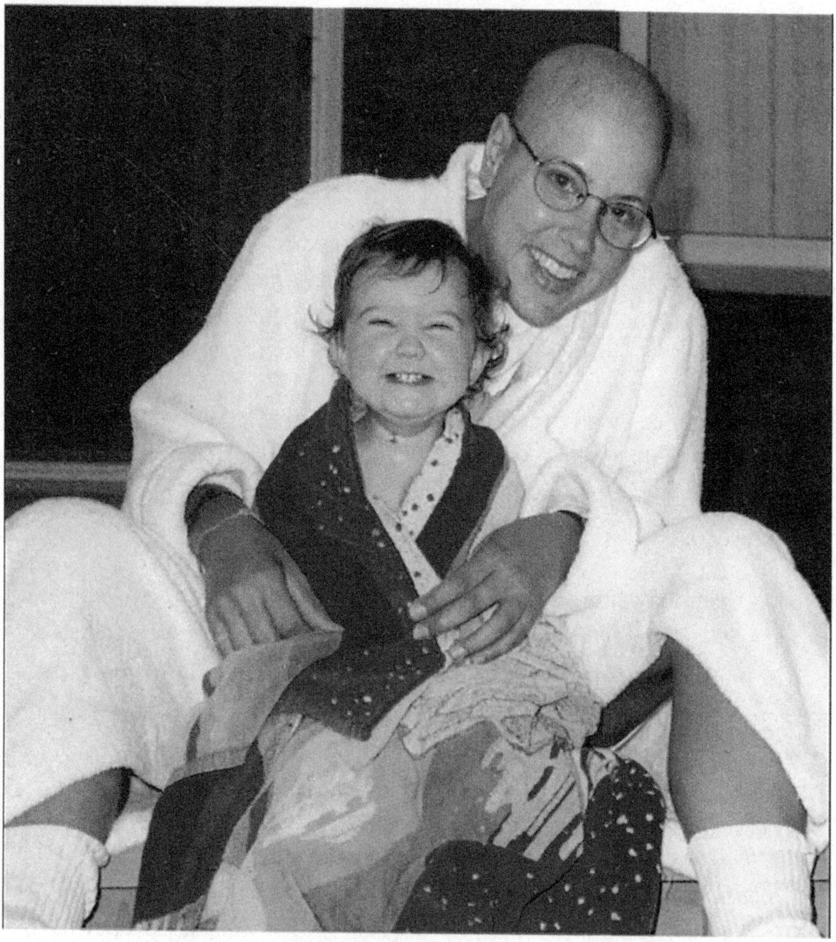

Jean LaMantia during her treatment

I called Canadian blood services and spoke to the nurse. I told her not to use my blood donation from the previous week. While I didn't have a diagnosis... the two options were both cancer and I didn't want that to be passed on to anyone through my blood. I've never been able to be a blood or bone marrow donor since.

Before I could see the oncologist though, I needed confirmation. The first step was a lymph node biopsy. In about a week, I had my surgery and a lymph node was taken from my neck, I must say, the surgeon did a great job, as that scar is barely visible today. Now, that lymph node had to be analyzed by a pathologist...

which was taking about a week. Once that was done, I was told I needed to have a CT scan with contrast medium.

I mentioned that my symptoms had started about seven months earlier. I think my immune system had done a good job of keeping the cancer in check, as during that time, I mostly felt tired, and I had this unusual symptom of radiating pain and numbness in my arm if I drank alcohol...which I just avoided doing, so I was able to continue living as usual despite having cancer. But...once I gave that blood donation...I don't think my immune system could keep up and the symptoms were progressing like wildfire.

It felt like my tumors were growing noticeably larger every day. I was experiencing night sweats to the point that I was soaking my pyjamas and I had to change them in the middle of the night. I was losing my appetite and my energy, and I was nauseous.

Drinking a litre of contrast medium is not fun at any time, but when you haven't drunk a litre of anything in a few days...it was pretty much impossible. Since I had just returned from a backpacking trip to Mexico and Central America, I was staying with my parents while I looked for my next job. They lived in a small town, and we had to drive to the nearest city – about 45 minutes away for the CT scan. But that drive had a lot of large hills.

Since I had to down the litre of contrast medium 1 hour before my appointment, that meant I had to try and drink that while nauseous, while going up and down hills in the car. I remember my mother saying, "hold onto it", "keep it down". I had to ask her to pull over a few times as I didn't think I could keep it in. I'm not sure I even managed to get a ¼ of it in...that was tough.

I did that scan and thankfully, the ride home was a lot easier, without the pressure to drink that massive amount of contrast medium. Now, it was just a waiting game...waiting for the results of the CT scan and notification of the next tests that I needed.

In the meantime, my lymphoma was having a field day in my immune-compromised, post-blood donation body. The tumors were growing quickly, and the lymphatic system was slowing failing. As you likely know, one of the vital jobs of the lymphatic system is to transport fluid from all parts of the body back to the circulatory system. But what was happening in my case was that the lymphatic fluid was being picked up by the lymphatic capillaries and transported up the central lymphatic trunks, but because of the massive and fast-growing tumor in the middle of my chest, that lymphatic fluid was not going into my blood stream, it was being dumped into my lungs.

I didn't know this was happening. All I knew was that I was getting short of breath and that there was a heaviness in my chest. When a few months earlier I was going to the gym every day and doing a one-hour step aerobics class followed by one hour of weight training, now I was having to catch my breath after one flight of stairs. I could only speak about 3 words before I had to take a breath. In short…I was drowning in my own body.

I remember hearing my mother's voice on the phone speaking with the cancer clinic, asking what else needed to be done before I could be seen. I heard her say, "yes, it's a new diagnosis, but she is going downhill fast", "just tell me what else she needs to do before she can be seen, she's not doing well." They told her that I still needed a bone marrow biopsy and to come to the cancer centre, but that I won't be staying and won't be starting my treatment, this is just for staging the cancer. My mother told me "pack your bag…even though they say this is just for the test, once they see you, I don't think they are going to let you go home."

She was right of course. They did do the bone marrow biopsy (negative thankfully) but once they saw this poor drowning person with her lymph slowing dripping into and filling her lungs…they said "we're admitting you, and we have one more test to do, a gallium scan, but we're not waiting, we're starting your chemo right away."

They admitted me and the next morning performed a thoracentesis. The thoracentesis was an interesting experience. I was asked to sit up in my hospital bed with my legs over the side and to place my arms over the bed table leaving my back exposed for the doctor. The doctor then placed needles into my back and I could feel the fluid draining out of my lungs. At this point, my water-logged lungs (or more accurately, my lymph-logged lungs) were experiencing air for the first time in a while and they felt like crepe paper and like I was getting more air than I could handle. I started coughing and couldn't stop, they put me on nasal prong oxygen which helped.

I remember turning around and glancing at what was removed and I saw two bottles of murky looking liquid. I later read my chart notes that said about 1200 ml of fluid was removed, which maybe doesn't sound like much, but it left a deep and lasting impression on me that there is a lymphatic system...it does some important stuff and if it's not working...you're...(I'll let you fill in the blank).

The next day I started on AVBD chemo – adriamycin, vinblastine, bleomycin, and dacarbazine. Since I'm writing this account for you today, you can guess that the chemo and radiation that successfully followed treatment my lymphoma. While that chemo regime was very rough for me, that's a story for another day.

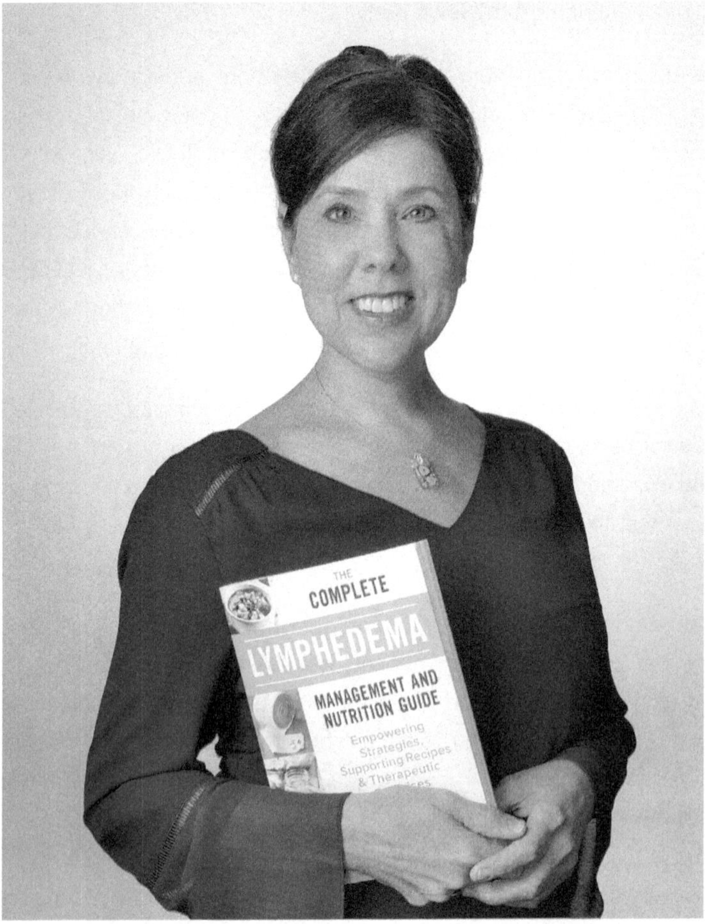

Jean LaMantia – The Complete Lymphedema Management and Nutrition Guide

Now, in my role as a registered dietitian, I work with other cancer patients and survivors as well as those whose lymphatic system is not working properly, no matter the cause. While my university education and subsequent clinical dietetic internship didn't prepare me for this, I've happily spent years reading every bit of research I can get my hands on about the role of nutrition in lymphedema and I've been able to share this with others and see real benefit. I'm happy to help people use nutrition therapy to make living with chronic lymphedema easier. Visit my website for further information *www.jeanlamantia.com* and follow me on Instagram *https://www.instagram.com/cancer_lymphedema_dietitian/*

TOP TIP!

I've seen how nutrition can impact lymphedema. One thing you can do for yourself, is to pay attention to what you eat and how it affects you. Changes you make to your eating can be very powerful tools in your lymphedema toolbox.

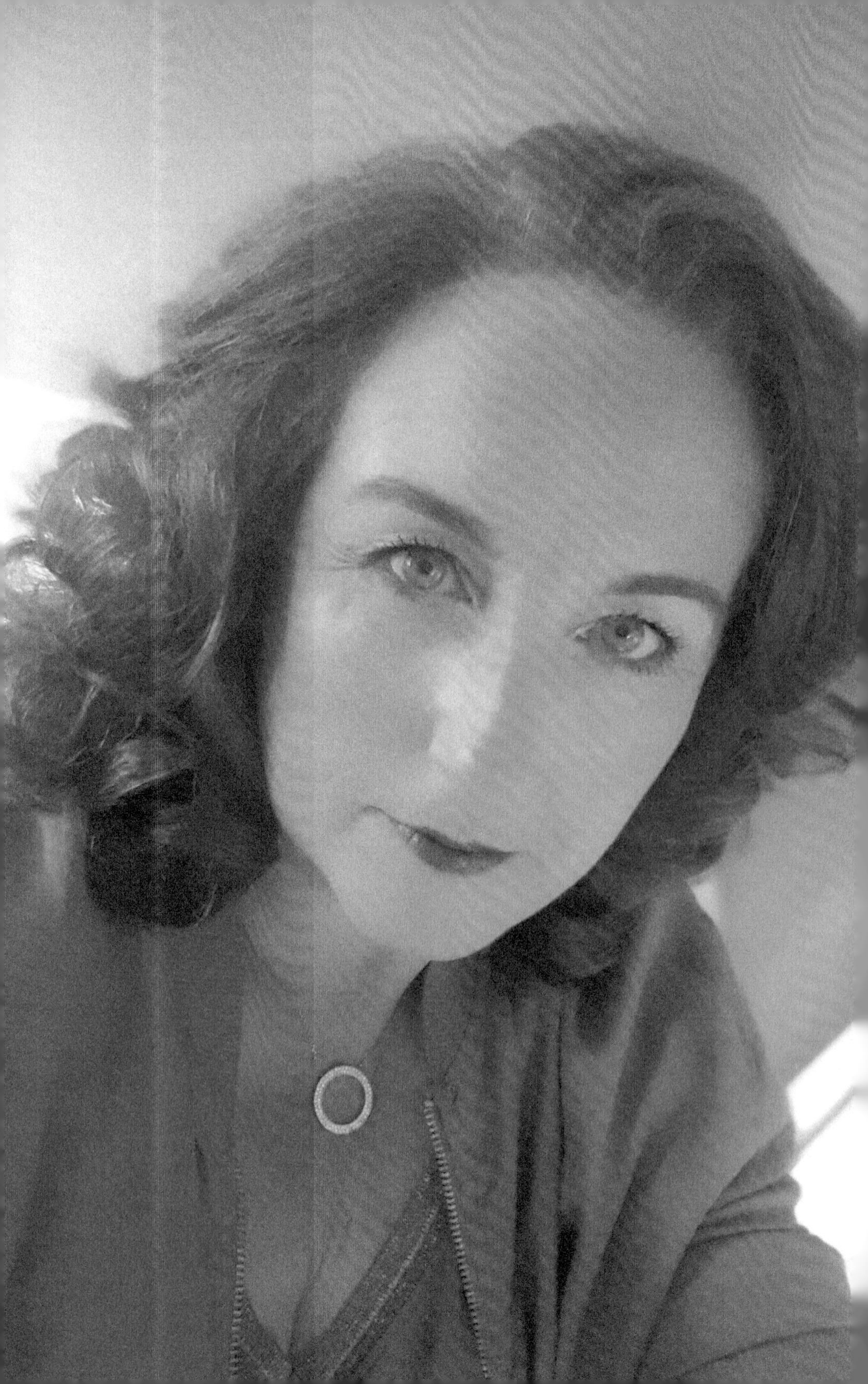

17

SIOBHAN HARRIS

> ***For me, physically and mentally I needed to have this surgery as I was not coping well with the size of my leg, or how it looked.***

I started to jot down notes on what I wanted to say in my chapter, sitting in hospital recovering from my first horrendous bout of cellulitis, a condition I had managed to escape since being diagnosed with lymphoedema. If you have ever had cellulitis you know how nasty it can be. It absolutely floored me and I ended up in hospital for 5 days on intravenous antibiotics (IV).

Anyway, I digress, I should start by introducing myself. My name is Siobhan Harris and I have bilateral lower limb lymphoedema, post cervical cancer and radical hysterectomy with lymph node dissection.

I am clinging onto the last year of my 40's, (I don't know why as my 40's have not been kind to me, it has been like a rollercoaster that you can't get off!). I am married to a wonderful man Karl and have three beautiful children, Ciara, Eimear and Saoirse. My passion in life is horse riding, a hobby I enjoy with my eldest two girls Ciara and Eimear. Saoirse's passion is archery. She informed me that horse riding was just not her thing.

When I heard the words "you have cancer", my world just fell apart. Everything went through my mind; Was I going to die?; How would I tell the children and my family?; Would I lose my hair (vain I know but everything goes through your head when you hear those words). I met with the Surgeon and went through everything that they had planned to do and went in and had my surgery quite soon after diagnosis. Thankfully, I didn't need chemotherapy or radium treatment and the cancer was contained, the dissection of the lymph nodes confirmed that it had not spread. I was so grateful that the cancer was gone at least then. I do not recall anybody mentioning to me to look out for the signs of lymphoedema as the lymph nodes had been dissected. Maybe they did, I honestly don't recall.

Roll on, about a year or so after my surgery, we were returning home from a fabulous family holiday in Florida, and I noticed my right foot was really swollen. It went down a few hours after landing. Looking back with the knowledge I have now gained about lymphoedema, this was obviously a sign that something was brewing. On my next visit with my gynaecologist, I mentioned the swelling in my leg to him and he said you have lymphoedema, you need to find a Therapist that deals with it and have Manual Lymphatic Drainage. That was the extent of his advice! There was a Therapist doing MLD in the same hospital as him and he never referred me to him. My journey into the world of lymphoedema and treatment or lack thereof as was the case, may have begun.

That day on returning home from hospital I was speaking with my mum, and I remember saying to her, "well it's only a bit of swelling at least I don't have cancer anymore". Oh my God, looking back how naive was I? Lymphoedema affects every aspect of your life. I saw a quote somewhere that said "Lymphoedema is like having a full-time job, but you don't get paid". To me that is exactly what it is like. I don't know about you but there is not one part of my life that lymphoedema has not affected, from the minute I get up until I go to sleep, it is there. Mobility, compression, skin care, garments, footwear, clothes the list goes on. I feel like I have to almost reinvent myself as clothes and shoes that I used to wear are no longer an option to fit over swollen limbs. Everything I do now is centred around my lymphoedema and whether it will affect the swelling. For me having lymphoedema is both mentally and physically draining. There is a constant battle not to let it get the better of me. I will admit there are lots of days when it does and I feel so depressed and angry, that the life I once knew has been robbed from me. These days are hard, but there are also good days and as time goes by hopefully the good days will outweigh the bad days.

In 2016, the news broke, through the courage and strength of the late Vicki Phelan (who I will eternally be grateful to for all that she did for the women of Ireland) that over 209 women, at that time, had had their cervical smears mis-diagnosed as being clear when in fact there were not. When this news broke, I received a call from my consultant to assure me that any smears that they had taken in the hospital while I was under his care were not part of this as they were tested in house and not sent abroad to be checked. I later found out that he omitted to tell me, that at the time of his phone call, he knew my previous 4 smears were misread and resulted in my cervical cancer.

I had just started a new job, well I returned to work for a previous employer, I was excited to be back catching up with old friends in a familiar place. Three days into my new job (I remember it so clearly it was a Friday), I got a call from one of my gynaecologist's team asking me if it was okay that a person from the HSE contacted me in relation to my cervical cancer. I was floored, I asked if I was one of the then 209 women affected by the Cervical Check debacle. The lady on the phone couldn't tell me anymore but that someone from the HSE would be in contact with me. I rang my husband in tears. I couldn't believe what I was hearing. So, I got a call and yes, I was one of the unlucky women whose smears were misread. I met with her the following Monday to go through the matter and then on the Wednesday I met with my Consultant to discuss the findings of the audit. Now, I am not usually lost for words, (anyone who knows me will concur) but that day in the Consultants office I was left speechless.

I listened to him going through the results of the audit and how my cancer was missed, and the smears were so incomprehensibly wrong. The icing on the cake was his confirmation that if they had read the smears correctly, I would not have needed to have a Radical Hysterectomy or lymph node dissection and, there-fore I would have not developed lymphoedema. My world fell apart yet again. Through the attempts of the HSE to save money by outsourcing the testing of the smear tests of the Women of Ireland, and their lack of due diligence, they have caused devastating life-long illness and some of the 221plus Irish Women affected by this Cervical Check debacle have needlessly lost their lives, leaving their families devastated.

I do feel guilty at times getting upset and depressed about my lymphoedema when some of the other women in the 221plus group have lost their lives because of the horrendous actions of the HSE and the Laboratories involved. Knowing that not only could my cancer have been avoided but that I would not have been left with a life-long chronic condition is a very hard pill to swallow.

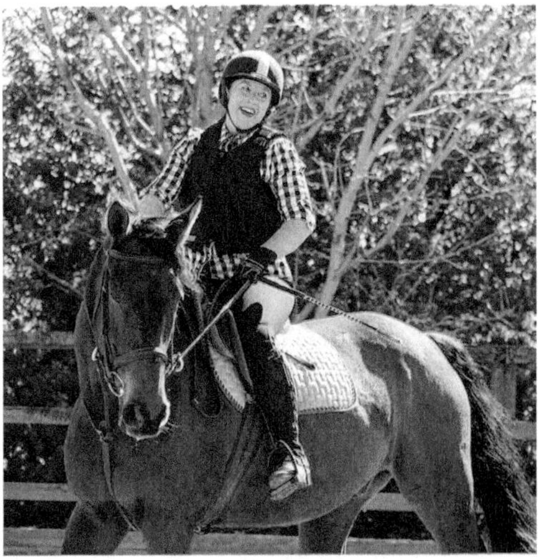
Siobhan Harris - Horse riding

Since being diagnosed with lymphoedema and knowing the circumstances that caused it and my cancer; in the first place, my life took a downward spiral of depression and loneliness. I didn't know anyone else with this condition. The first time I had MLD and compression bandaging I cried so hard, I couldn't accept that this was my life from here on in. I didn't want to go out, didn't socialise, missed family occasions because I couldn't find clothes to fit over my leg or shoes to fit my swollen foot. Even the one thing I loved to do horse riding was affected; I was terrified I would fall or get a kick from my horse, and I would hurt my leg. I no longer knew who I was. Lymphoedema can be a very lonely place. Reaching out for support did not come easy for me as I am usually very bad at asking for help. I knew that I could no longer do this on my own and I needed to get help. Over the last few years through research and reaching out to others with this condition I have met many wonderful people with the same condition, in addition to fantastic Therapists and suppliers, only too eager to help and support me on my journey with lymphoedema. Ireland unfortunately has a lack of support for lymphoedema. However, I will say that it is improving, slowly, I will admit, but it is improving and that can only be a good thing. I started to reach out to, and search for treatments other than M.L.D for my lymphoedema as I was not dealing well with the size and extra weight that I was carrying in my right leg at the time. It has now unfortunately spread into my left leg, groin, and stomach.

I've been to the Wittlinger Clinic in Austria for complete CDT (Complete Decongestive Therapy). This clinic is fantastic! You are able to concentrate fully on your treatment with two sessions of MLD per day, exercise classes, gym, pool etc and the most fabulous scenery and walks to get that lymph moving. I have to say the results were great and I got a good reduction in my leg. However, once I returned to normal life the swelling came back. Like I said earlier, having lymphoedema is like having a full-time job but you don't get paid! It never gives you a minute.

As time was moving on, I was not dealing with my Lymphoedema well. Most people still saw the smiling happy Siobhan, but those who knew me well, my family and friends and my amazing work colleagues knew otherwise. I decided to look into other options of treatments that were available. I came across the Oxford Lymphoedema Practice in Oxford, England. I researched them and made an appointment to speak to one of the surgeons. I had a Zoom call with Professor Dominic Furniss, an amazing man. We chatted for I'd say over an hour. He went through my history and discussed in-depth the treatments they do and what he felt would be the best course of action for me. I went over to Oxford later that year to meet with the Surgeons and have some tests carried out, prior to deciding to go down the surgical route. At the same time, I had an appointment with Professor Mortimer to get his expert opinion on my condition too. Both Professor Mortimer and the surgeons in Oxford concluded that having Liposuction for lymphoedema was the best option for me, at that time, because MLD and bandaging was not going to reduce the volume in my leg any further than it was. For me, physically and mentally I needed to have this surgery as I was not coping well with the size of my leg, or how it looked. Also having to carry that extra weight in my leg was affecting me badly, and I was not doing well.

So, in December 2021 I went ahead and had the surgery. It is a hard surgery and recovery is tough and painful. However, I knew it was worth it when I looked at my legs and they were almost the same size again. It really helped me deal with lymphoedema on a better level and I will be eternally grateful to the team in

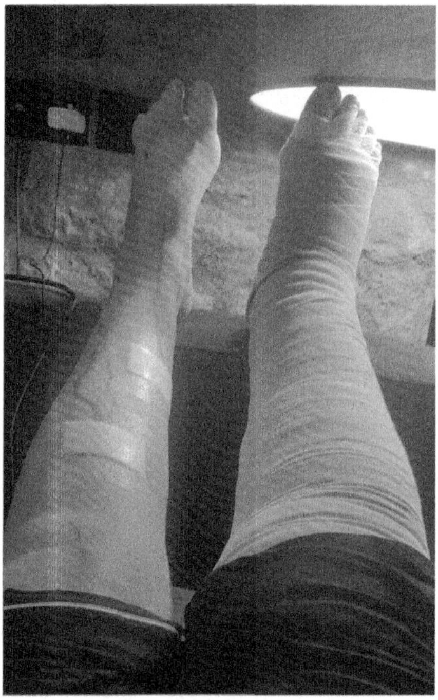

Siobhan Harris - After LVA Surgery

Oxford Lymphoedema Practice for their expertise, professionalism, and friendliness. They certainly played a huge part in helping me live my life with lymphoedema and not let lymphoedema totally consume my life.

While the surgery did make a huge difference to the size of my affected leg, it doesn't take away from the daily maintenance required to keep on top of lymphoedema. As I said before, lymphoedema is like having a full-time job, but you don't get paid. My daily routine includes self-manual lymph drainage or dry brushing in the mornings. Skin care after my shower as it is so important to keep your skin in good condition. Then it's straight into compression garments which for me are toe caps, made to measure class 3 tights, and a class 2 stocking on my right leg also. A lot of armour and an absolute nightmare in the heat! I am currently taking a break from work so in the mornings I will go for a walk, horse riding or maybe a swim, anything to try and keep active so that the lymph fluid can be pumped and try and get it moving. I will also do a bit of deep breathing when I'm relaxing which is great for moving the lymph fluid also. During the day I will rest and raise my legs to help reduce any swelling. Movement is key for lymphoedema as unlike the circulation system the Lymphatic system does not have its own pump, so you have to move to pump the lymphatic fluid. At night time I either sleep in the garments, bandage or use a night time garment. I think it is good to try as many different compression products as you can to see what works best for you. I also have a manual lymph drainage session once a week and in between sessions I have a compression pump at home that I can use. There are also days when I might not even have the energy to get a walk in and I will just take it easy on those days and listen to my body and relax. This is also important for your self-care.

Now as you know if you have this condition, it is not easy, you have good days and bad. Hopefully as time goes by and you learn to deal with this condition and reach out to get the help that is out there, the good days will outweigh the bad. We are a special community and everyone I have met throughout my journey with lymphedema so far, has been more than willing to help, give advice, share their tips on how they manage on a daily basis. So, don't be afraid to ask for help, we know what it is like to live with lymphoedema, so we get you and your struggles. We understand. I think without the support of my family and many friends (you know who you are and all the free therapy sessions you gave me) I would not be where I am today. I don't think I will ever forgive the HSE and the US Laboratory for causing this, but I am learning to live better with lymphoedema. I started the Lymphoedema Toolbox to help others in Ireland and worldwide to source the help they need and let them know about new garments and clothes etc, that are available to help make living with lymphoedema a little bit easier. Unfortunately, I had to put that on hold for the time being. It is just on the back burner for now. Hopefully by the time you are reading this my legal case has been sorted and I have started to close that chapter of my life and begin a new happier one and maybe when the time is right The Lymphoedema Toolbox will be back bigger and better. We will see.

If I had one top tip to share with you that has helped me on my journey it would be self-care, you need to mind yourself first, do what you need to do to look after you and your Lymphoedema, then you can look after others. Remember you can't pour from an empty cup.

Love and Light

TOP TIP!

Self-care is important! Look after yourself and your lymphoedema, then look after others.

Remember, you can't pour from an empty cup.

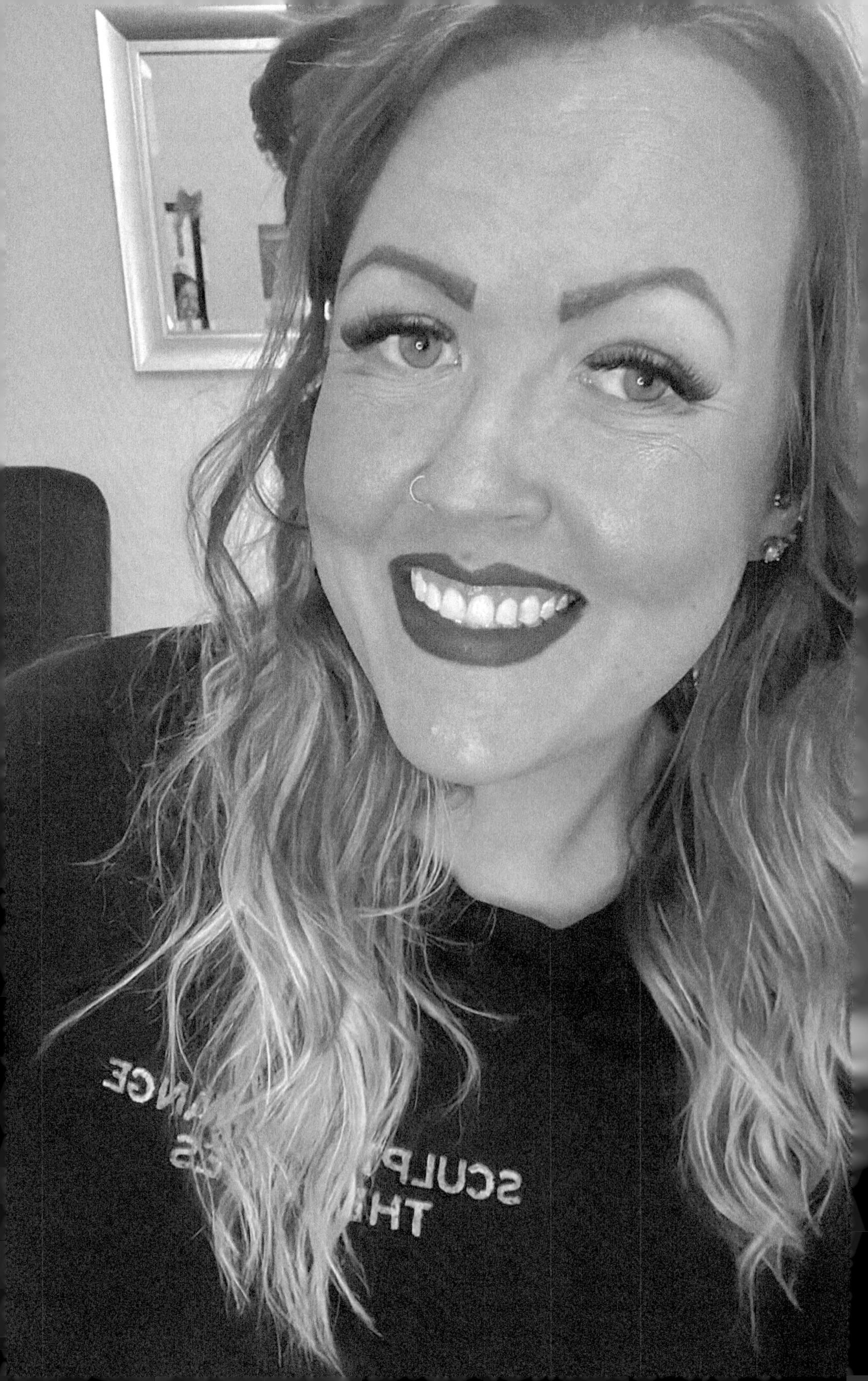

18

KAREN WINDSOR

If I didn't lose any weight and if I didn't try and do something about my health, I was going to end up in a wheelchair. This gave me the biggest wake-up call of my life!

My story is unusual because it started with surgery that turned into secondary lymphoedema. At the time I was already a very big girl but that comes later, when you find out that I had an underlying illness of lipoedema pretty much my whole life but lymphoedema was masking it.

In 1999, I had a quite serious fall down some stairs and I indented my left leg and didn't think anything of it at the time. The following morning, I woke up and had pretty bad bruise and went to Accident & Emergency (A&E) at the local hospital. I was told to 'take some painkillers and you'll be fine.' I think it was 10 weeks later when coming home after a night out with some friends, I had what looked like half of a football on top of my left shin.

I was quickly sent to hospital where they said that I had got an infected haematoma which is a bruise that has gone inwards rather than outwards. I ended up with an awful lot of fluid that had collected around my bone, and it was causing what they thought could be an infection. I had to have it lanced and filled with gauze and this was a procedure I had done without anaesthetic as it was too late, and it had to happen there in then. I was later discharged and was told to come back regularly for intravenous antibiotics, but they didn't change the gauze in my leg which then became infected.

I was sent to my doctors who took one look at me and sent me straight to A&E, where I was quickly put on gas and air to have the gauze cut out. I then had a skin graft to graph the area, which was kind of successful, although it did take about six months to heal and I did need to have a lot of dressings. However, something always felt off or not quite right about the recovery.

Fast forward to 2005. I was at work one day and the area of my leg became itchy, and the skin had started to lift, which was quite scary. I quickly got in contact with my doctor's surgery and told them what was going on and they told me to go straight to A&E, which I did, where I was told that the area could be infected. I decided to go and see a private consultant who said I needed to have a skin flap repair. So, I went and had a consultation for a skin flap repair, which involves cutting out all of the bad area and then they pull the skin over and stitch it up. In doing so, my lymph was hit and we didn't know that until after that particular surgery. I was at home, and I happened to be standing and I look down and, already being a big girl because of the lipoedema which we didn't know about at the time, my legs had started to seriously swell, and it became quite scary. I went straight back to the hospital and luckily there was an Australian lady who was in the physio department and knew about bandaging. She said straightaway this is lymphoedema. I had no idea what she was talking about. She decided that we were going to bandage it all up and they quickly got in contact with Saint Catherine's Hospice, which is a place where they had a lymphoedema clinic. I was quickly sent to St Catherine's Hospice. I was very lucky that these things happened quickly for me.

I was then sent to St Georges Hospital in Tooting, London to see Professor Mortimer which was probably one of the most important appointments I've ever had in my life. At nearly 26 stone, I went to see Professor Mortimer with an open wound on my leg and with what I didn't know at the time was lymphoedema. He made it very clear to me that if I didn't lose any weight and if I didn't try and do something about my health, I was going to end up in a wheelchair. This gave me the biggest wake-up call of my life! I didn't know how I was going to get from A to B and hearing that woke me up like you wouldn't believe! Prof Mortimer said we have to start a course of treatment including bandaging and compression and so I spent three years in a layer bandaging and compression to bring the swelling under control.

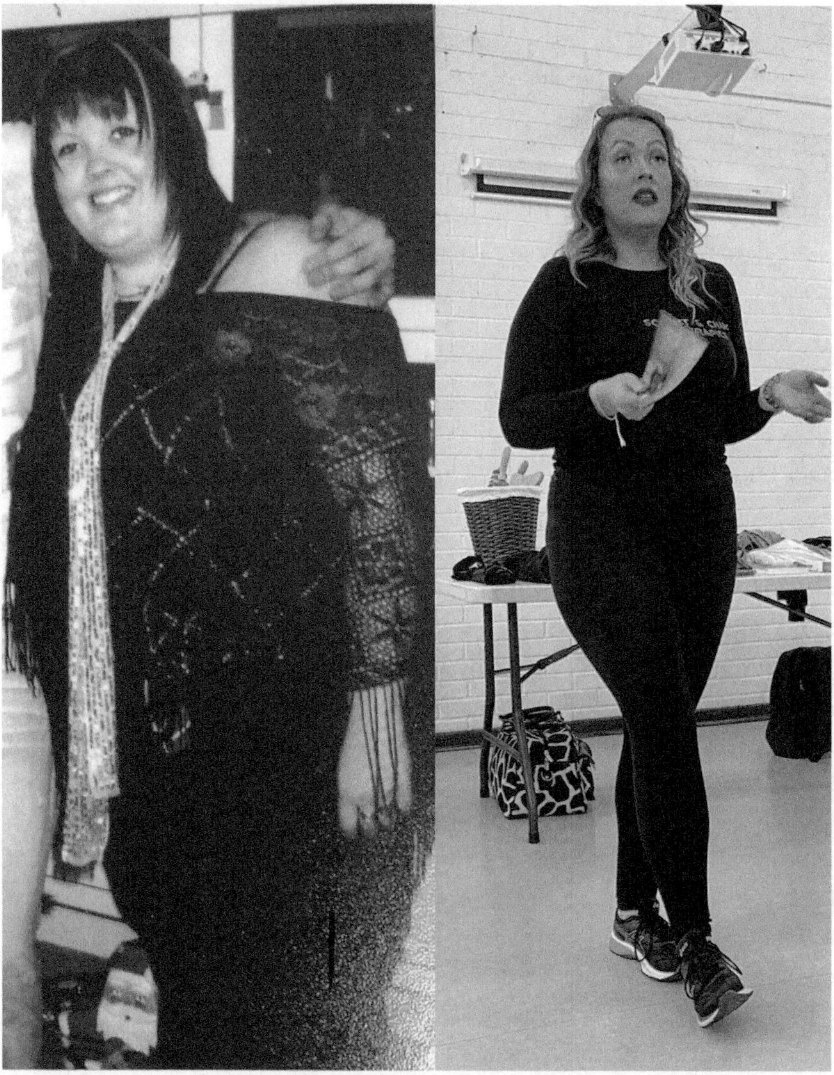

Karen Windsor - Before and after

I wasn't diagnosed with Lipoedema until 2015. During the 10 years from 2005 to 2015, on top of dealing with the lymphoedema, the experts I had over 30 surgeries to try and close the wound and had so many different dressings and so many different vacuum packs that I ended up on crutches. At one point, I had to wear leg braces as my joints were seriously weak. This was one of the hardest Times in my life! Now, I look back and realise that this was teaching me everything I needed to know to go forward with what I've done today.

When you are going through some of the toughest times in your life, you can be difficult to see the light at the end of the tunnel.

It can feel like the whole world is coming down on your shoulders and you're being punished for something, or you're being torn apart for something. I now realise that everything that I've been through was to build me up to become the strongest light force I can be and to help others in our community going through similar circumstances to what I had suffered.

During the following 10 years I spent focusing on nothing more than lymphoedema, I was in a bad place in my head. I wasn't a very nice person to be around and I was angry a lot of the time. I was also confused a lot of the time and I had developed some bad habits. I wasn't the person that I wanted to be. Then I started to see a lot of improvement with the lymphoedema, but I knew there was something that wasn't right with me. I had met a few people who had lymphoedema and one of them was Amy Rivera and another lady called Sarah and another called Elle. This was all on social media and these women with lymphoedema were able to lose weight by looking after their lymphoedema on a daily basis. However, I couldn't, and I knew something was going on with my body, but I wasn't sure what and I kept questioning this from about 2010. I kept questioning, do I have Lipoedema and then in 2015 I finally got the answer. I knew I had already got it and the experts said yes, the lymphoedema was under control and it was masking lipoedema. So, I then had a new fight I had the diagnosis of an abnormal fat connective-tissue disorder, alongside having LYMPHOEDEMA. To say that I wasn't in a good place is an understatement! The diagnosis continued to come for another couple years and in 2016 I was diagnosed with fibromyalgia and chronic fatigue and Dercums disease. That was another big blow because I was slightly smaller and because fluid and inflammation was under control, and I was now having to deal with this abnormal fat cell. I then realised that my joints just were not working, and I was in many different leg braces. I was unstable and would fall and my joints would bend backwards. I was in and out of hospitals seeing different consultants who would immediately put my issues down to my weight, I then saw a rheumatologist and they sent me to a musculoskeletal hospital where I had tests for hypermobility. The Beighton score came back that I had a nine out of nine score for hypermobility and EDS better known as HEDS, plus a diagnosis of osteoarthritis in the left knee.

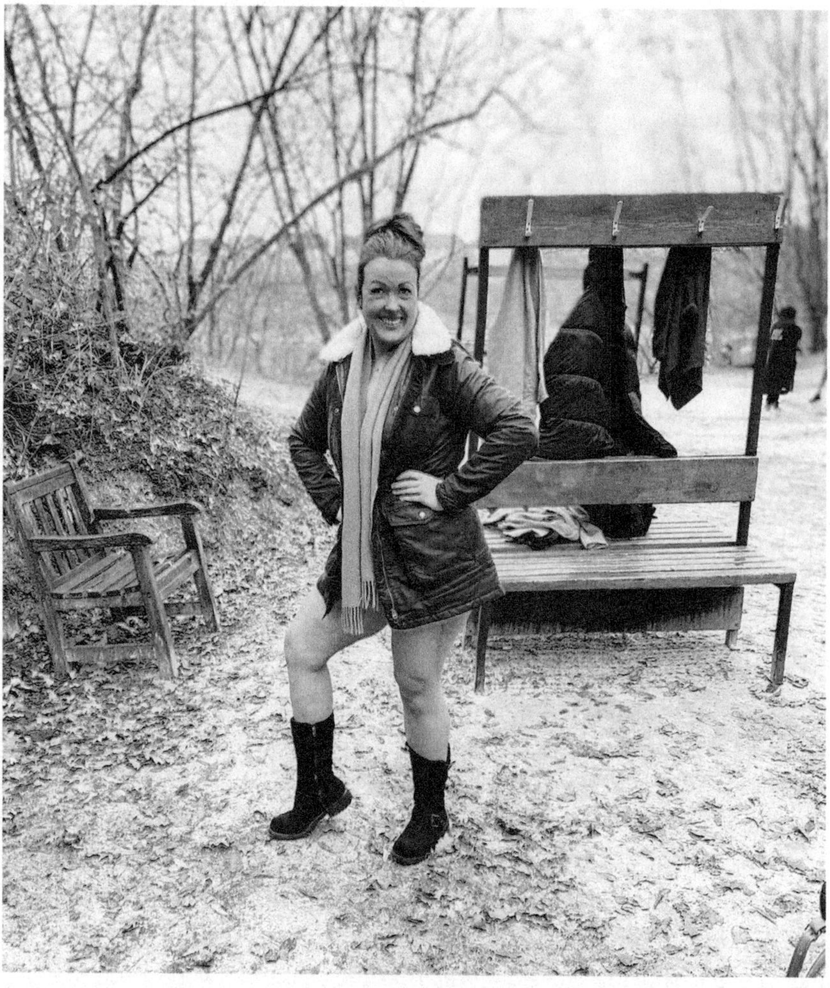

Karen Windsor Lake Swimming

Can you imagine what that does to a person and how it makes a person feel? I was lost! I didn't know how to live. I didn't know how to get my life back on track, so I asked for help from the NHS for a treatment for lipoedema and I found all of this information out after I joined the charity Talk Lipoedema, which saved me. I am now a trustee for them.

I went through rigorous consultations with consultants, and I had to have photographs taken in x-ray and put all of that together with my doctors who applied for approval for this particular surgery, which could've changed the outcome of how I'm living with my joints. I am convinced of this, however, I was turned down for the surgery under the guise of it being cosmetic and they were extremely apologetic and knew that this was going to make me very fragile and upset, but there was no funding as it was deemed as cosmetic.

So, I've hit a wall again and didn't know where to turn so I went to see a private consultant and the cost of the surgeries that I needed was just completely out of my price range. There was no way that I would be able to afford it all and I couldn't ask anybody to do this for me, so I hit rock bottom. I got to a point where I was like what's the point? I am going to be living with this for the rest of my life. I'm probably going to end up in a wheelchair. I'm probably going to end up needing assistance, so what's the point? I can tell you when you hit rock bottom you can only go up and circumstances lead to me getting very angry with all of this and thinking that this was how my life was going to be.

No chance! I'm taking my life back every little step and I have listened to advice, and I have been taught many different things, and slowly I build myself back up. However, I didn't just build myself back up, I changed my whole life! I changed who I was, I changed my identity, I became my true authentic self, I decided I'm not going to be a victim anymore. I'm going to build a business and I am going to help people in the same circumstances and I'm going to help them change their lives! Nothing or no one is holding me back. This is never going to happen again and that's exactly what I've done. I've built Sculpt & Change Therapies a successful holistic clinic focused on conservative treatments dedicated to lymphatics connective tissue and hormones and helping thousands in person, online, and in workshops. I have clients that fly from around the world to see me. I have clients that travel from all over the UK, and it is because they can relate to me, because I have gone through it and come out the other side. I will continue to come out the other side and I will continue to be the light in the dark that they are going through.

Join my Instagram page @kaztalks for regular posts to help you move forward. Visit my website for more information about my treatments at *www.sculptchangetherapies.com*.

TOP TIP!

Wear your compression garments and dry brush for 2-3 minutes per day. It's cheap and easy and so effective.

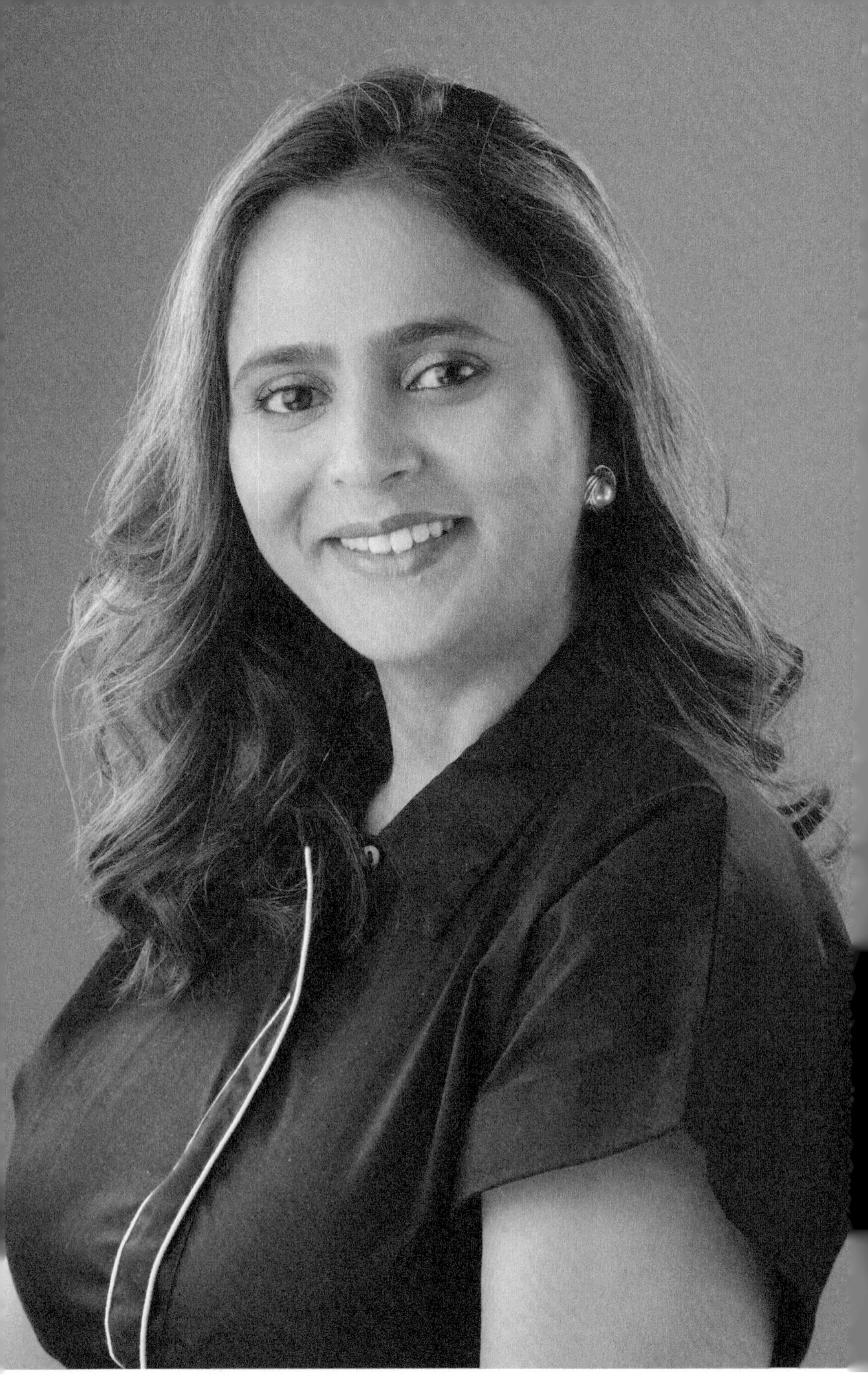

19

KRUTI KACHALIA

> ***Realizing that love must be found within oneself before seeking it externally, I took charge and decided to educate myself about my condition.***

Admitting that falling in love this time wasn't love at first sight, my journey from wishful thinking to acceptance has been far from easy. It all began with my ignorance of the term "lymphedema" and the realization that I had acquired it as a result of axillary lymph node dissection during my breast surgery. As a member of the medical fraternity, I felt embarrassed for not being informed or counseled about the lifelong consequences that awaited me, surpassing even the challenges of a harsh tumor diagnosis in Secondary Lymphedema.

The bubble of my obliviousness finally burst when I reached a critical stage of lymphedema and couldn't find proper Complete Decongestive Therapy (CLT) in my vicinity to manage it effectively. I underwent the initial decongestive phase at a renowned hospital, considered a knowledge hub for such conditions, but after five weeks, I saw no improvement at all.

At that point, I found myself pondering, "What comes next?"

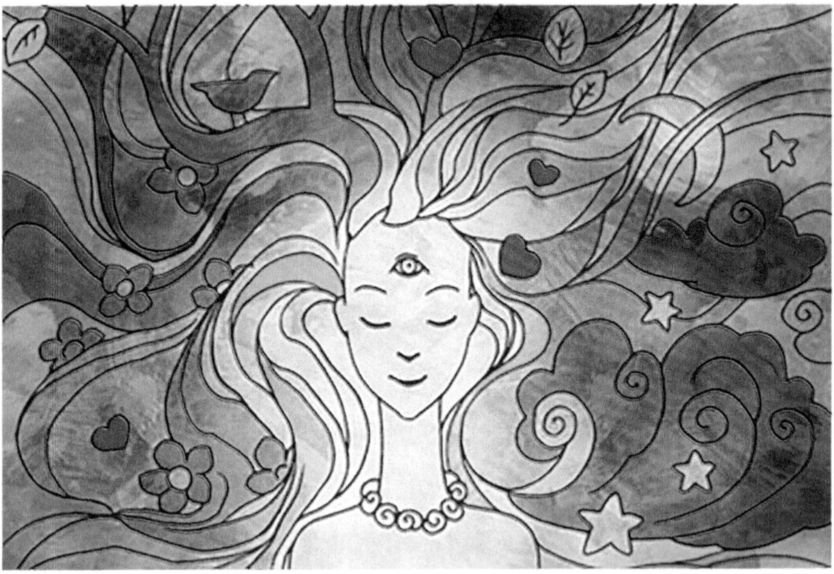

Self-Education and Awareness Is Self Empowerment

Realizing that love must be found within oneself before seeking it externally, I took charge and decided to educate myself about my condition. As a doctor, it may seem unconventional to rely on internet resources, but I took my first step by turning to Professor Google—the vast realm of the internet.

I delved into available information and started reading extensively. To my surprise, I discovered an incredible wealth of help and knowledge through social media platforms. It introduced me to a global community of fellow lymphedema sufferers, where I came across blogs and connected with the right people at the right time. Among them was Amy, whose blogs proved to be a valuable resource for my self-lymphedema management. Through Instagram connections, I learned self-manual lymphatic drainage (MLD) by engaging with certified lymphedema therapists (CLTs) and other patients.

This journey allowed me to gain a profound awareness of lymphedema, the knowledge that was not easily accessible in India. The experience motivated me to take on the challenge of becoming a CLT myself. When I had the opportunity to enrol in a course conducted by a reputable training school in India—something quite rare—I seized it. Despite being a secondary lymphedema patient, my background as a surgeon allowed me to participate.

Throughout the training, my trainer was astonished by how I had educated myself primarily through the right social media channels, using them as invaluable sources of information and guidance.

When Life Throws Lemons at You - Squeeze Them into Lemonade!

This became my guiding principle when I discovered the world of yoga, even before I started exercising, practicing manual lymphatic drainage (MLD), or using compression bandages. I embarked on a journey of yoga, which proved to be instrumental in maintaining my condition throughout the years, even when I was unaware of the concept of compression.

Through focused asanas (postures) and breathing techniques, yoga became a form of Pranic healing for me. It not only nurtured my physical well-being but also imparted valuable life lessons of self-acceptance, inner peace, and happiness. It was through this holistic practice that I experienced a profound sense of clarity—an understanding that when you love and accept yourself, people and the world around you naturally adapt to it.

Best Version of Myself

I underwent a remarkable transformation, evolving into a revitalized 2.0 version of myself—overflowing with enthusiasm to learn and adapt to the ever-changing challenges of life and lymphedema.

Just as there are days of consistent lymphedema management and occasional flare-ups, life itself is a series of ups and downs—nothing remains constant. Embracing this realization liberated me from the victim mentality that often engulfs us as patients.

Gone were the days of concealing my condition or camouflaging my arm with loose-fitting garments! Instead, I developed a heightened sense of fashion-consciousness and skilfully incorporated my lymphedema into my personal style, ensuring both comfort and elegance.

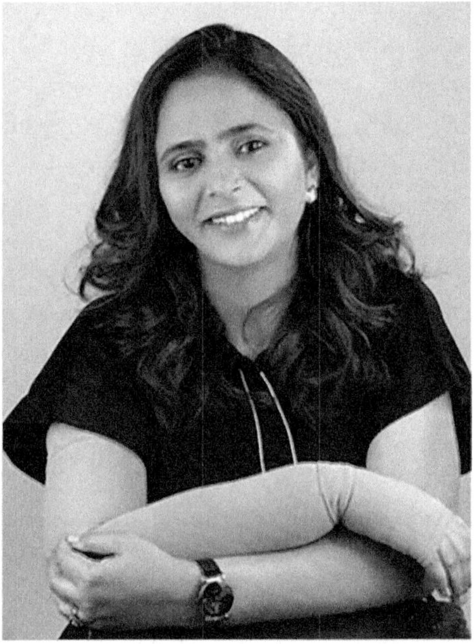

Kruit Kachalia - Best version of myself

Few Lessons Learnt in This Journey

1 **Pamper Yourself:** Pampering is not limited to spa treatments or retail therapy; it's about dedicating time to self-care and nurturing oneself like a baby. Despite its challenges, this lesson has been invaluable to learn.

2 **Better Time Management:** While juggling work, kids, and family, it's crucial to prioritize and allocate dedicated time for lymphedema care without fail. Although I'm still working on mastering this skill, whenever I've achieved consistency, I've experienced the remarkable benefits. Consistency is the master key!

3 **Life is Beyond Sulking Over Lymphedema:** Sharing experiences with our community and educating others is liberating. By raising awareness, we can eliminate the stigma surrounding lymphedema, encourage early diagnosis, and ensure appropriate treatment. Additionally, the demand for quality medical care will increase, necessitating more trained doctors in this field.

4 **Educate-Innovate-Educate:** Proper education plays a vital role in developing innovative approaches to make lymphedema management more enjoyable. This includes fun workout sessions, engaging collective activities with support groups, stylish and comfortable compression garments, creative dressing techniques, and more.

5 **Ask for Help:** Be open to accepting help and offering it to others, especially if it contributes to self-care and overall well-being. I received tremendous assistance from social media blogs and even patients whom I had never met before. Help can come in various forms—emotional, mental, physical—and if it helps anyone bounce back, it's worth embracing. Hence, I am ready to stand anywhere in support of my tribe now.

6 **Stay Elevated:** Both in Posture and in Life: Maintain good posture physically, but also strive for an elevated mindset and outlook on life. This entails staying positive, embracing challenges as opportunities for growth, and constantly seeking personal and professional development.

TOP TIP!

By incorporating these 6 lessons into my journey, I have discovered profound wisdom and a renewed sense of empowerment.

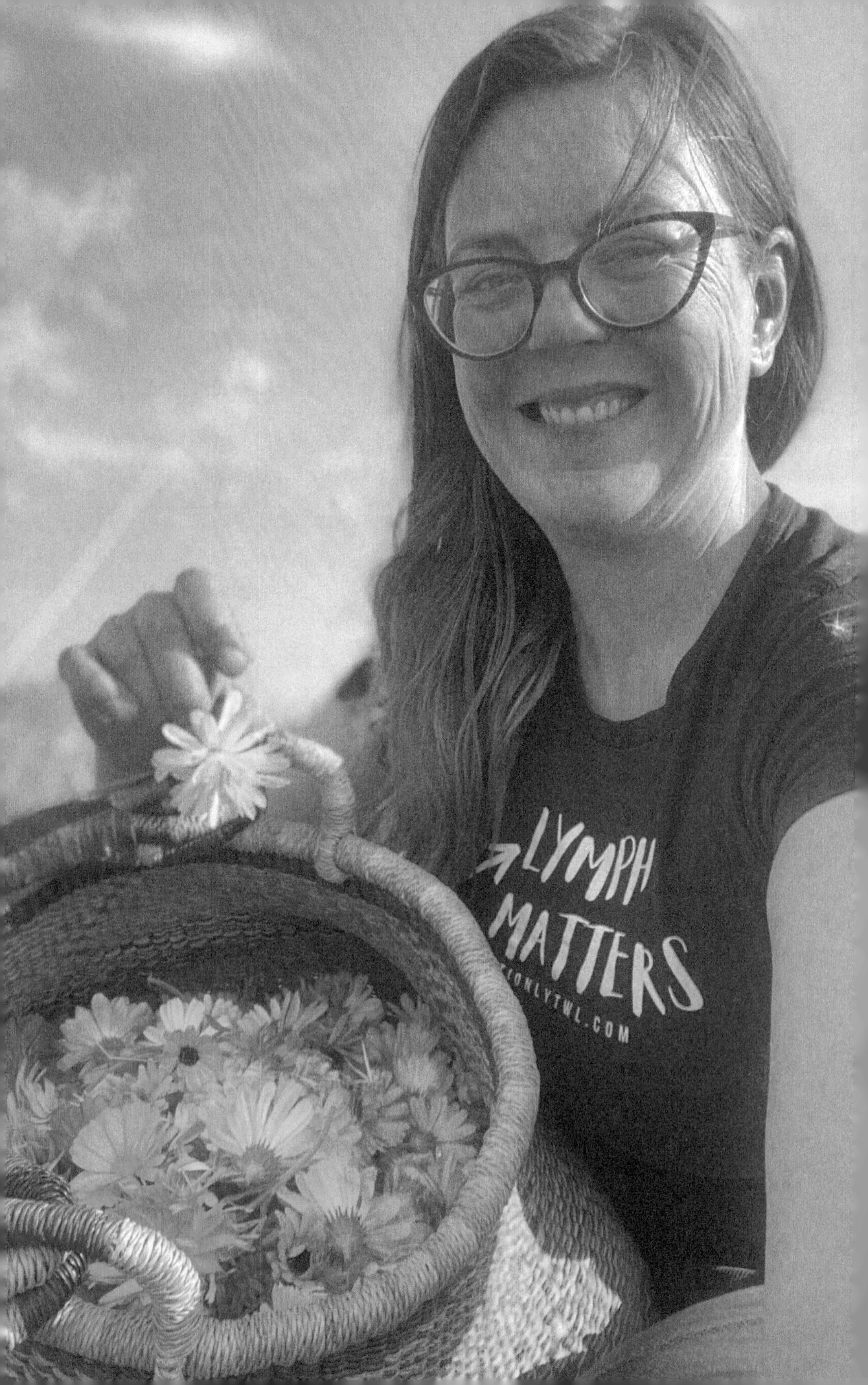
LYMPH
MATTERS

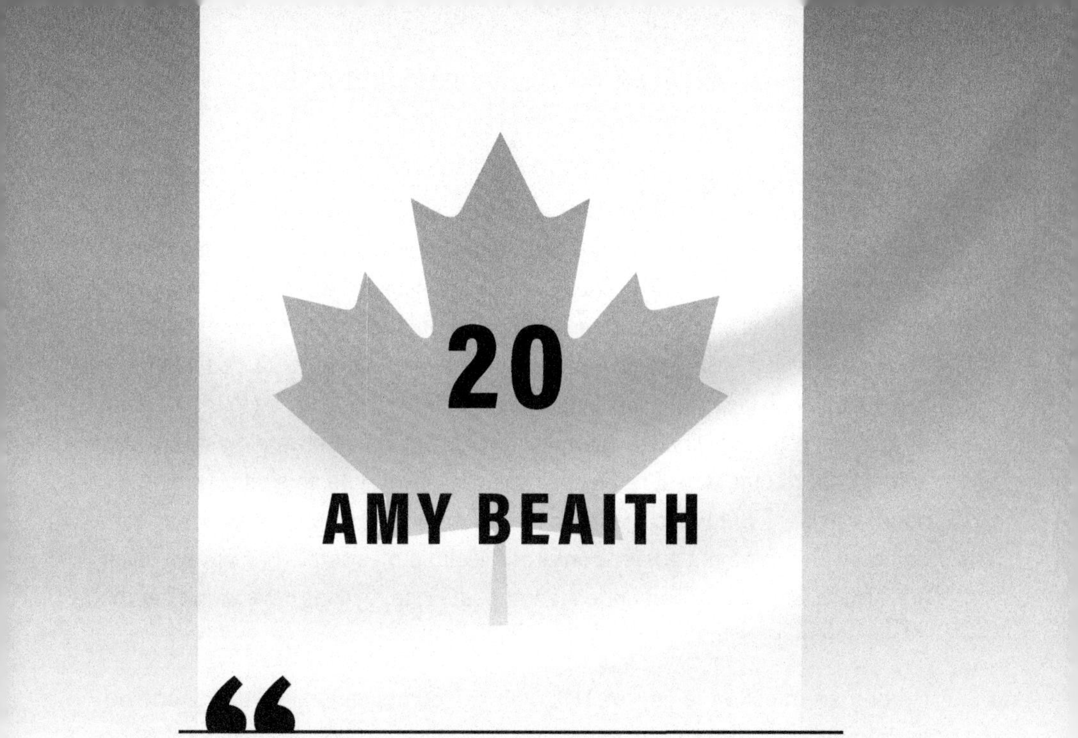

20

AMY BEAITH

> ***I'm healthier now than I was in my twenties and it's thanks to advocacy and daily self-care.***

I've lived with Lymphedema since I was 5, but I didn't learn to manage it well until less than 10 years ago. After a tragic series of events, I realized I had to become my own advocate and began to take my power back through self-care. At the time, I was struggling with recurrent cellulitis infections, watching my lymphedema progress like a speeding train that wasn't stopping, living in fear that I might lose my legs someday. To today, where I no longer live in fear of infections, and I rarely get them. I'm healthier now than I was in my twenties and it's thanks to advocacy and daily self-care. When I was younger, I wish someone would have told me how much power I can have over my life through lovingly caring for my body holistically. I'm grateful for my Lymphedema because it has taught me how courageous, strong, resilient, and creative I can be. The most important thing I have learned is to be my own advocate and share my voice so that no other lymphie has to struggle like I did and to remember that our bodies are beautiful, exactly as they are, deserving of our love and care now and always.

Let me tell you my story. As I lay on a hospital gurney with a severe cellulitis infection up my entire right leg. I was in excruciating pain. This was my 26th such infection in my legs since my early 20s, tears were flowing down my face, and I was sobbing uncontrollably as the IV antibiotics soaked into my veins with relief and sadness. It all started 36 hours before, when I had gone to the Emergency Room (ER) with a suspected infection, remembering previous advice I had been given. 'Amy, with your history of infections, don't wait, get yourself to the hospital as quick as you can.' I'd had so many, I knew how to spot the warning signs, even before I got the trademark red rash. I was seen by the doctors after waiting 8+ hours at the ER, but without a red rash, I was given no medicine and was sent home. I was dumbfounded and confused. Health professionals had always taken my infections seriously and understood I could lose my legs if we didn't get the infection under control!

Getting an infection is one of THE WORST complications of Lymphedema. It can affect you physically, mentally, spiritually, and socially, leaving lasting effects that can be harder to manage. In those 36 hours, waiting for antibiotics, years of hard-earned progress was vanishing before my eyes. The effects of self-care habits of wearing compression daily, exercising regularly, eating healthily, were vanishing. My right leg was more than 2 times its original size. My shoes didn't fit, nor did my pants. In that moment, my leg and spirit felt so heavy, but there was also a feeling of anger brewing below the surface. Why had I not been listened to? Why had I been turned away with my history of infections?

The antibiotics had literally saved my legs and my life many times and I was very grateful for that. However, my life felt like it was becoming a series of recovery sessions from one infection after another, barely making it a year before I would succumb to another even stronger one. The strong antibiotics were leaving my skin, gut, and mind in disarray with more rashes, food intolerances, and anxiety each time, and I began to wonder if they might not be strong enough one day. If my body might get too used to them and they would stop working.

That day I broke down on the hospital gurney with nurses staring at me wondering why I was crying so hard. I knew in that moment I had to do something different. I began to hear a voice inside me that said ***'there has to be more than this, there has to be another way'***.

I let my anger fuel my drive to find answers. To help me see that this was not my whole story, nor was it the end of my story. It was only part of it, and that my life was going to get so much better!

I had a young family, with two beautiful girls and a husband I love dearly. So, I dug deep and listened to the voice inside me that said ***'there has to be more, there has to be another way'***. When I said this over and over to myself as a mantra, a calmness began to wash over me.

In order to change my outcome, I knew I needed to change my approach to my Lymphedema care and ask different questions. I had to open up my eyes and find new to me examples of people thriving with and people treating Lymphedema.

"When you change the way you look at things,
the things you look at change."

—WAYNE DYER—

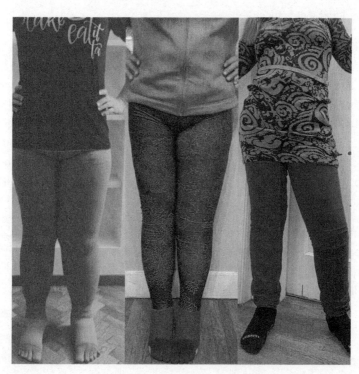

Amy Beaith - The Process of Progress

As a former Health Librarian, I used my research skills and began searching for anything I could find. Lymphedema is a world-wide phenomenon, so it was time to connect with some lymphies around the world and learn about their experiences.

Little by little, I found people thriving with Lymphedema. Many of us with Lymphedema can feel very alone. Having a community can make such a big difference mentally, physically, and emotionally. When you see others coping with what you are coping with you can feel seen and understood, accepted in new ways. You find people that can help create solutions together and motivate each other. You share ideas and experiences on what helped you bounce back after a set-back, lymphie jokes, and even lift each other up when someone *just can't lymphie that day.*

It was in this community, that I first learned about Lymphatic microsurgeries. In some countries, these surgeries had been offered for 30+ years, but it was largely unheard of here in Canada. Why? I was sceptical at first, thinking what do you mean surgery? We aren't even supposed to get a cut on our limbs! How can surgery be safe for us?

I also began to include stronger self-care habits based on insights I was gaining from other lymphies in my online community. Looking back, during this time, it was a lot like throwing spaghetti at the wall to see what sticks, in order to find out what was helping my Lymphedema! I didn't have a framework for Holistic Lymphedema Self-care to follow like I do now. I tried adding/changing exercise, meditation, yoga, foods, journaling, women health circles, and different compression techniques. I tracked my changes and slowly started to get a sense of what my body needed, but also what a Lymphedema self-care framework could look like for myself and others!

Later in 2017, I went to France to have a Lymphatic MRI, and meet Dr Corinne Becker to see if I was a candidate for lymphatic microsurgeries. We talked about the fibrotic tissue load that I was carrying from having had so many infections. Each infection had laid down scar tissue in my body, that was making it harder for my lymph to flow. Removing some of that could reduce my risk of infections substantially. This could be a game changer for me!

Nine months later, it was time for surgery! From the moment I arrived, I felt cared for and knew I would be in good hands with Dr Becker and her team. I had

Suction Assisted Protein Lipectomy (SAPL) and a Vascularised Lymph Node Transfer (VLNT) in my left groin. I'd had Primary Lymphedema in my left leg since age 5, and in my right leg since age 30. They took out 2.5L of fibrotic tissue and successfully implanted a VLNT, which was harvested from my left rib cage area.

Recovery from these surgeries is no joke! I could barely walk from my bed to the bathroom the first day after the surgery. My leg was covered in bruises and oh so tender! But my leg was so much smaller and lighter, and softer, so, it lifted my spirits despite the pain I was in. Each day I got a little a bit better and before you know it, I was back home in Edmonton where I continued my post-op recovery.

Having the surgery healed me in more ways than I was expecting. My first session back for Manual Lymphatic Drainage (MLD), my massage therapist couldn't get over how much smaller BOTH my legs were! We measured both legs and were astounded to see that my right leg had mirrored the drop in volume and had changed over 2L in size on its own!

Our bodies really are amazing! I'm glad I trusted my intuition and challenged myself to find out what other treatments were out there and pushed hard for the ones that felt right for me. It wasn't easy challenging the Alberta Health Services, writing letters, making appeals, only to lose in the end. But I pushed on anyway and paid for the surgery on my own. The belief that 'there has to be another way' guided me to this moment. If I hadn't had that traumatic event, watching my leg balloon with an incredibly strong infection, unable to get the medication I needed soon enough, I might not be where I am today.

There are valuable lessons in all our experiences, if we are willing to see the whole picture.

One of the incredible benefits of the surgery was that my tissue was now softer and more responsive. Self-care became easier and was more effective on my pain and swelling. My surgery journey wasn't over yet. In 2021, I had SAPL surgery again. This time on my right leg and here in Alberta. It was a success and both legs benefited again! I was so fortunate and grateful.

These surgeries have been an important tool in my Lymphie toolbox. I believe, they truly work best with strong self-care before and after. My Lymphedema is well controlled today because I take an integrative approach to my care, employing the best of what western medicine can offer me as well as holistic self-care practices and lifestyle. I wish someone would have told me years ago how much ease and calm I could have in my daily life by being my own advocate and by taking control of my self-care. Using my voice, and implementing small, simple, daily self-care habits have stacked up to profound, lasting change.

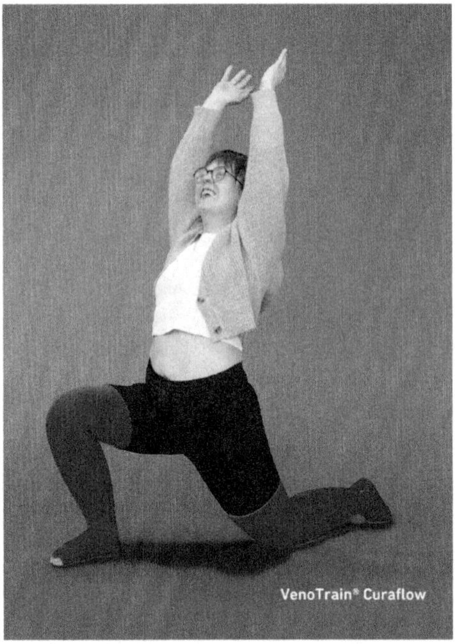

Amy Beaith - Stretching her beliefs.

What is Lymphedema Self-Care?

Over the years, I've developed a framework of Lymphedema self-care, which came partly from those throwing spaghetti at the wall sessions, as well as from Herbalism and Ayurveda medicine teachings. It was in Ayurveda that my eyes were opened again in a new way because of how important they believe the lymphatic system is to our overall health. Our lymphatic tissue is the first tissue formed in the body and affects the health of all the other tissues. Ayurveda states that our inner waters are living and involved in every single cellular process in the body. Imagine what your life could look like if you saw your lymphatic system this way too?

Ayurveda translates from Sanskrit to mean 'the science of life.' It focuses on building daily and seasonal self-care routines with the rhythm of nature. Learning and implementing its teachings has allowed my self-care to shift towards more holistic, responsive, intuitive and loving ways of caring for myself. I became less focused on finding fixes and solutions that could make my Lymphedema better and began to see that rituals and routines could support my overall body to stay in balance, which would in turn improve my Lymphedema too.

One simple teaching from Ayurveda that you could try today, is building a healthy sleep routine. In Ayurveda, everything has an energy to it, including the time of day. The hours between 10pm-2am is detoxification time when the organs of the liver and kidneys are most active. One of the key roles of the Lymphatic system is to remove waste from the body. Sleeping before 10pm can set your body up well for the next day by giving your body time to detoxify. This reduces your overall inflammation load, strengthens your immune system, and helps you get the most our of your experiences by giving your body time to integrate them into your physical and energetic bodies. When you have a compromised lymphatic system, ***this one little step of going to sleep early is free and it can make a big impact on your swelling and overall health***. Give it a try and let me know what you think!

My life with Lymphedema looks so much brighter today than it did less than 10 years ago. With a supportive, self-care routine and lymphatic microsurgeries, I have remained infection-free in my left leg for over 5 years now and only had 3 minor infections in my right leg. This outcome is something I couldn't have imagined a few years ago. Our human bodies are capable of more healing and transforming than we sometimes realize!

I now teach other folks with Lymphedema how to build holistic self-care routines through my unique framework that combines Yoga, Ayurveda, and Herbalism. I'm also a Lymphedema ambassador for Bauerfeind Curaflow. Lymphedema self-care doesn't have to feel like a burden or a chore that you dread. I'm here as your Lymphie self-care coach with 40+ years of experience living with Lymphedema. The daily self-care habits you chose, stack up over time to have profound effects. You have more control over the state of your Lymphedema than you think. You can take your power back through self-care. Learn to listen to the whispers of your body so you don't have to hear the screams. I would love to help you shift from surviving to thriving. It is possible and it's in your hands.

For more information visit my website www.lymphwell.life and follow me on Instagram @lymph.well

TOP TIP!

The hours between 10pm-2am is detoxification time for your lymphatics. Like a nightly reset button. Going to sleep early is free and can have a positive impact on your swelling and overall health.

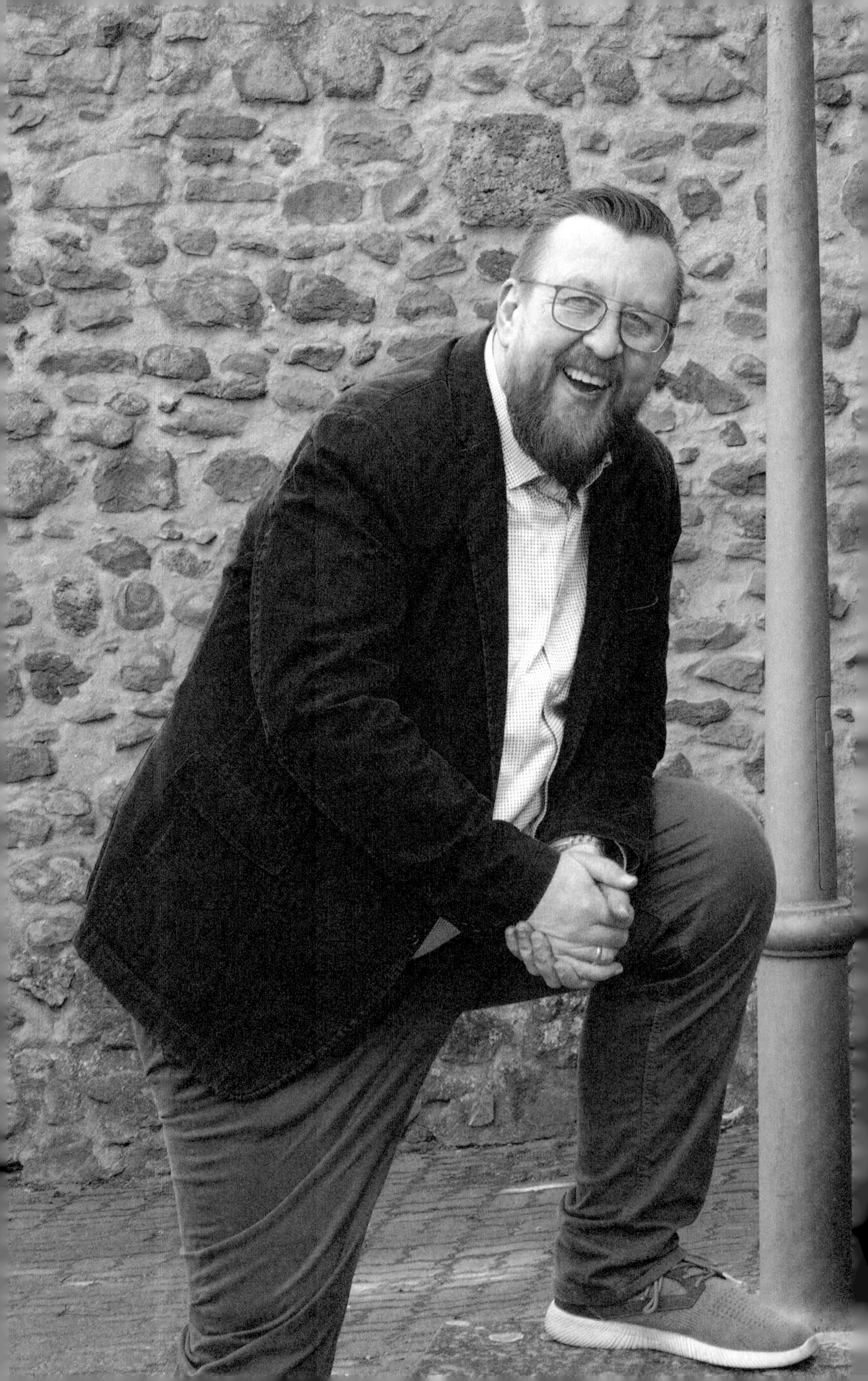

21

JÜRGEN JAKOB

> ***Consistent wearing of compression stockings from early in the morning until late in the evening was advised.***

I was born on a Sunday, March 22, 1964 in Giessen (Germany). A Sunday child! The childhood was relatively inconspicuous, I was stocky, but not fat and preferred to run around in shorts.

What I did not know at that time, is that I had a hereditary condition called lymphedema from my father, which broke out in puberty, at the age of 13. I was on a big vacation at my grandma's farm, about 200 km from home. I felt listless that summers day, I was pale, and my groin lymph nodes hurt. I had to lie down. Over the next hour, I developed cellulitis – colloquially named erysipelas – on both legs. This started with chills and fever and my legs became red and hot from the toes. The calves were especially affected.

The fever climbed very high to 40 degrees, so the doctor was called. The country doctor, however, did not know this symptom and prescribed cold compresses.

Fortunately, we already had penicillin tablets, which provided some relief after a few hours. In my legs there was water retention, which did not regulate even after the erysipelas subsided. Swelling in both legs was evident.

After a few days back home, I presented the symptoms to my family doctor, who diagnosed lymphedema. I have two brothers, an older brother and a younger brother. The older brother did not inherit the hereditary disease, but the younger brother did. Over the years, lymphedema appeared in him as well. Our father had passed it on to his boys in the hereditary material. He himself had only worn compression stockings in the course of his life, but also very often fell ill with erysipelas.

I could not come to terms with my thick legs and sought answers in all kinds of examinations. I also visited a special clinic in Bad Nauheim. It was a specialized clinic for heart diseases. So the doctors suspected that me, at the time only a teenager, had heart disease and that the water could be expelled. Under painkillers – sugar cubes with drops – I was anesthetized and from the toes of the foot a red rubber garden hose about 3.5 cm wide was placed around the toes and wrapped with force applications the water from the toes over the back of the foot, ankle and calf, in the hope that the water was expelled and no longer accumulated.

What was probably not known at that time, was that this method was counter-productive for the lymphedema because this probably damaged the lymphatics even more than they already were. It was inevitable that I too would have to wear compression stockings. I was given Class 2 stockings which went up to my knee. At that time, people still spoke of "rubber stockings", which was actually a sanitary article for older women. So, of course, as a teenager, then 16 years old, I felt ashamed.

Together with my family doctor, I found a specialized clinic in the Black Forest, which was located directly on the highest point of the Feldberg in Breisgau. The Feldberg Clinic in Altglashütten lay dreamily between lush meadows and dark fir trees. There were a lot of patients here, most of whom suffered from secondary lymphedema. They were mostly women who had had a mastectomy and the lymph nodes under the armpits had been cleared out widely. This resulted in the formation of a thick arm. Rarely were there men as patients – and if there was a man, it usually meant surgery in the groin or abdomen was the cause. Primary lymphedema was rarely found there.

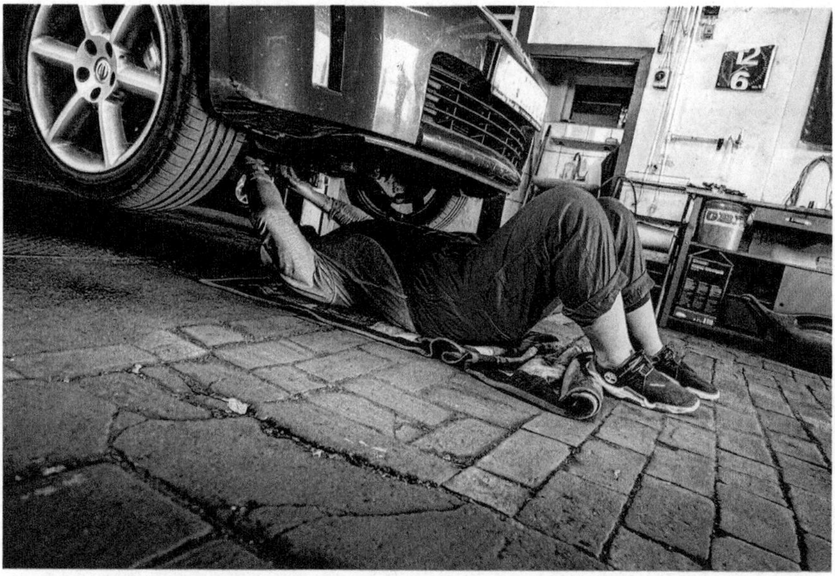

Jurgen Jakob firing on all cylinders. Image courtesy of medi. Photo: www.medi.de

At that time, Prof. Dr. Földi and Dr. Asdonk were still working together in the clinic and researching the clinical picture. Back in 1981, everything was actually the same as today: lymphatic drainage – 2 times a day and wraps from the toe to the groin. The elastic bandages softened the tissue very quickly and stimulated the lymph flow. I often had to go to the toilet during the lymphatic drainage, that's how strong the effect was. Also, my heart and kidneys were examined. I was taken to a clinic in Freiburg to find out whether my thyroid gland was the problem or whether I had heart disease. Here they examined the person holistically – from the tip of their toe to the top of their hair. Here I was, as a young man, hospitalized for about three-quarters of the year. Finally, the compression stockings were fitted to measure and given to me for further treatment. There were also many lectures on lymphedema. Prohibitions and suggestions – the focus was on weight reduction even then. Absolutely forbidden were sauna sessions, sun and warm vacation countries.

Consistent wearing of compression stockings from early in the morning until late in the evening was advised and 2 to 3 times a week lymphatic drainage, involving the whole body for 60 minutes each session.

The doctor advised good skin care, so that no injuries would occur, disinfectant after the swimming pool, so that no athlete's foot could form, hygiene like an operation. If possible, wrapping with elastic bandages was also recommended to patients, because no other therapy went beyond that.

Advice on a healthy balanced diet, rest and recreation, avoidance of stress and anger was also given to the patients to take home.

I came here again and again for rehab until I had somehow integrated it into my everyday life. I had a severely disabled pass issued by the pension office where I received the 50% GdB for an indefinite period of time.

The school time was a spit-route run. I dreaded every sports lesson or swimming class. I tried to hide the compression, which at that time was only beige in color, and I also tried to hide my thick legs. It was especially unthinkable to come to gym class without shorts and in the locker room of the swimming hall all the boys were lined up and there was no exception. Somehow, I managed to run into the water and then it was time to rest until it was time to go back to the locker room. When it came to indoor sports, I was allowed to be released from attending, by my doctor.

Another challenge was getting to know women, especially when going on a date. At the end of the evening, my next concern was about undressing, and I had to hide my worries about my stockings and thick legs. In the summer it was the time to wear shorts and I always ran around in long pants, even at 30 degrees. Sometimes, I used to get strange comments from other men.

I experienced huge burden when I had a permanent partner. I made it clear to every woman that I never wanted to marry or have children. Of course, this was due to the hereditary disease, which I did not immediately reveal to every woman. With my current wife, the two of us discussed the topic at the university clinic in Giessen in the genetics department. Here I actually learned more about lymphedema, which was well known there and so the questions could be answered. I was particularly interested in whether I could actually pass on this disease to my children. I found out that each partner passes on 50% of their genetic material, but only men were affected in my family. The doctors discussed with us how to break this chain to give birth to girls. They explained how we could do this, which had to do with taking the woman's temperature. However, they decided against this method, which was to produce children on command. They just let it happen and I am pleased to say we have two children, both female.

In both children lymphoedema has not broken out and was not apparent until today. According to the Genetic Institute, there are other clear criteria to detect lymphedema: that is a double row of eyelashes – the eyelashes grow very finely on the eyelid and secondly, the two toes next to the big toe. These are slightly connected, it seems as if they are twins. This is what they are called in medical jargon at the medical supply stores. In fact, me and my younger brother both had these hereditary characteristics.

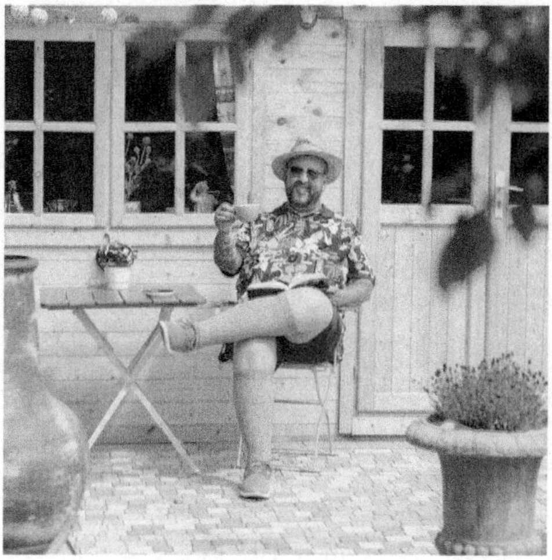

Jurgen Jakob avoiding stress.
Image courtesy of medi. Photo: www.medi.de

To this day, I recognise that it is important to avoid stress, because every time I have a high level of stress, erysipelas (cellulitis) breaks out. Usually, it can be treated at home if penicillin is taken immediately in high doses or administered by injection. If it takes longer, for example because no medication is available, the erysipelas becomes severe and I have to be put on a drip in hospital. Usually, I'm in hospital for about 14 days. To try and counteract this, I take homeopathic globulins that really prevent erysipelas.

Today, I am open about my illness and even model for medi, a well-known compression stocking manufacturer. I am self-confident with this disease, occupy talk shows and happy to pass on knowledge about the subject.

TOP TIP!

I recognise that it is important for me to avoid stress, because every time I have a high level of stress, erysipelas (cellulitis) breaks out.

medi

medi®, a family-owned premium compression therapy company, caters to the needs of lymphedema therapists and patients through a hands-on approach to develop products and solutions to create positive outcomes.

medi embraces the opportunity to support advancing knowledge in the lymphatic world. Our shared extensive experience in the marketplace serves the overarching needs of our community by driving high-quality products, education and efficacy of treatments that will push successful outcomes for all.

We have identified core challenges within the lymphatic clinical landscape and have developed unique products and educational support to address:

- Accuracy & fit
- Efficacy of treatments for diseases
- Challenges of compliance

How Do We Help?

After a major earthquake hit Haiti in 2010, medi created a non-profit called medi for help to provide aid quickly. While the need has been focused on the poverty-related, neglected tropical disease lymphatic filariasis, we've also had the opportunity to help other communities in need, such as Camp WatchMe, the first and only summer camp in North America for children between ages 5 and 17 who all have lymphedema.

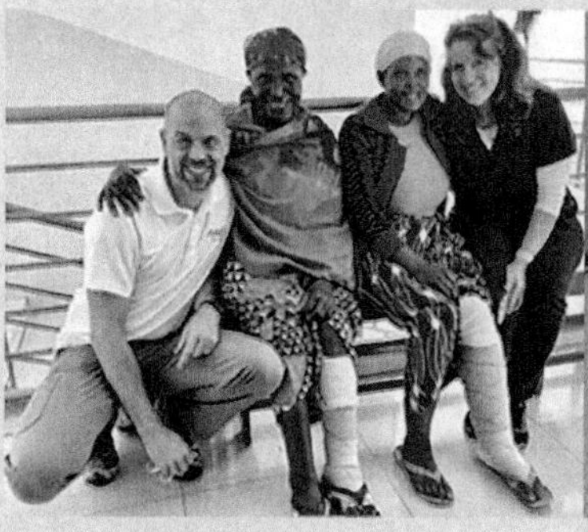

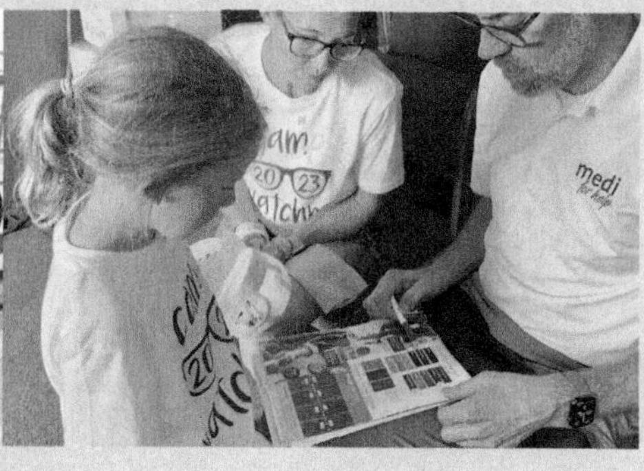

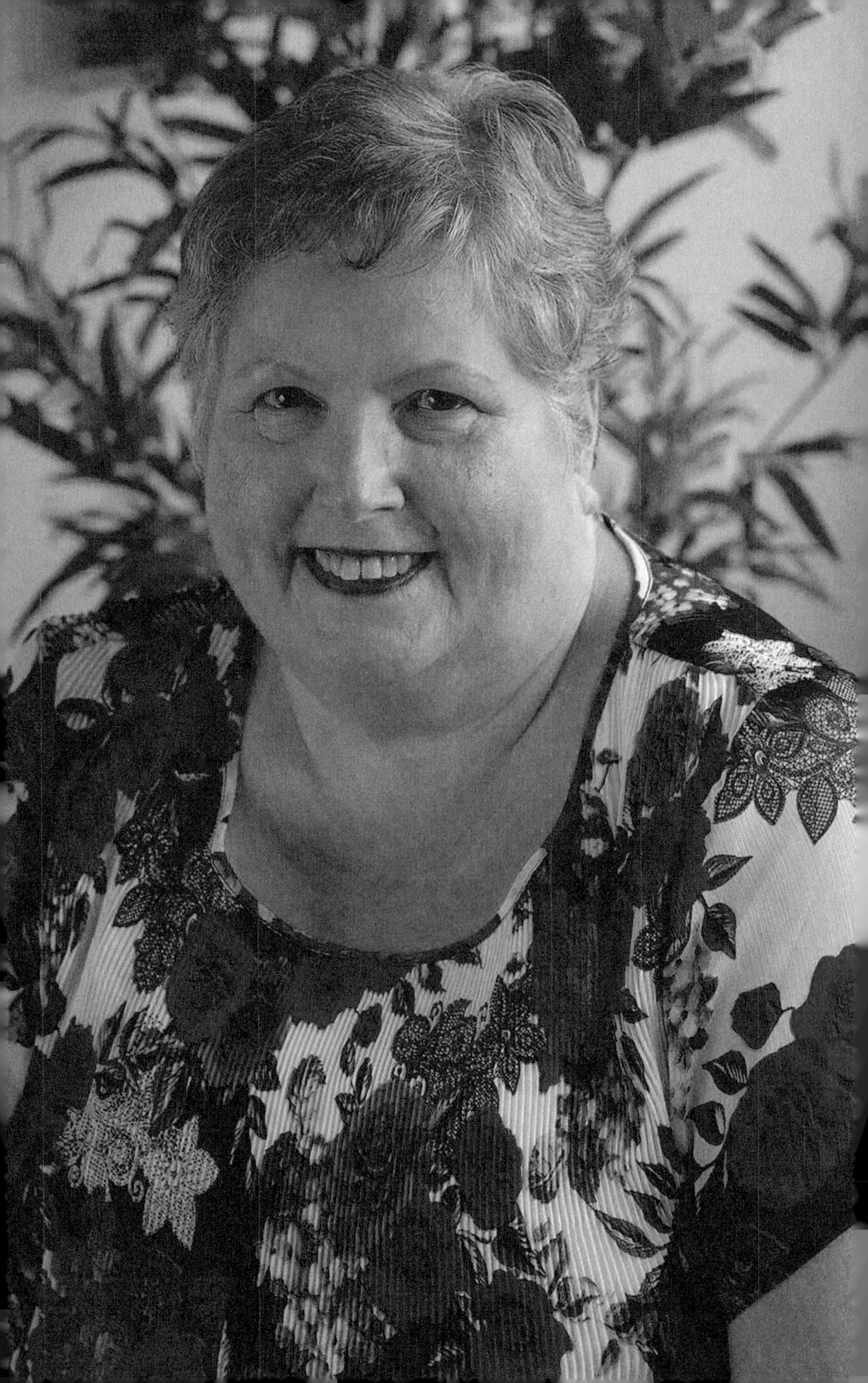

22

GAYNOR LEECH

I believe you can accomplish whatever you feel capable of.

Those first few months after my diagnosis of lymphoedema my life was filled with negativity as everything was focussed on the 'lifelong' and 'incurable.' Not once did I hear that lymphoedema could be managed or treated. I felt doomed. Anger transformed into a desire to better not just my life but also to share my story and, in a tiny way, the hope that if I could save just one person from experiencing what I did, it would be worthwhile.

I received a letter late in 2010 inviting me for a routine mammogram. In the UK, women between the ages of 50 and 71 who are registered with a GP will be invited for Breast Screening (Mammogram) through our National Health Service (NHS).

Breast screening checks use X-rays to look for cancers that are too small to see or feel. I have previously experienced benign breast lumps, all of which were removed. I wasn't unduly concerned, after all it was just routine and my appointment at the breast clinic went without a hitch. A few days later our planned holiday to Turkey with friends went ahead and we had a lovely holiday that still holds lots of fond memories.

While we were away, our boys had been watching over our house and had gathered all the mail and placed it on the coffee table for when we got back. A letter with the designation NHS was at the top of the stack of mail, and I realised that something was amiss. The letter was an invitation for additional testing.

I am forever grateful for that routine mammogram; it saved my life. My breast cancer was not a lump it was in the tissue, and it would not have been found without the mammogram at such an early stage. To all intents and purposes my long-term prognosis was good, I had breast conserving surgery to remove the offending tissue and 15 days of radiotherapy to mop up any remaining cells.

At my first appointment, in May 2011, with my Oncologist after the radiotherapy treatment, I was in a positive state of mind. I had several questions prepared and asked her when my breast might go back to normal. As it was beetroot red, hard, and uncomfortable, but thankfully I had no burns. Her face turned white as said quietly "You have lymphoedema" my response "lymph what". This I repeated three or four times. It was then she said, "We must get you and urgent appointment at the hospice". My head was spinning at this point, and at first, I thought I had missed or not been informed of something regarding my disease. Yes, I did think that I was going to die.

At that time, I thought a hospice was somewhere you went for palliative care. However, hospices in the UK run other services, including wellbeing services, community services and lymphoedema clinics.

To give it its full name my diagnosis, breast, and posterior chest wall lymphoedema. I do not experience the same problems finding clothes that fit, as many do, because of wearing compression. My problem was with bras, and it took me four years to find one that I would be comfortable with. The cup size of the bra becomes problematic if you have breast lymphoedema. By the end of the day, I would need a cup size that was four times larger on my affected side than I would in the morning due to lymphoedema swelling. The unaffected side stayed the same. Now, as long as I maintain any swelling by self-lymphatic drainage, it is rarely troublesome. I was not given compression by the clinic, but I have since been able to wear the Comfiwave breast band, which is fantastic because my swelling is at its worst during the summer due to the heat.

The hospice provided me with eight years of excellent care, which included manual lymphatic drainage (MLD) and I was taught to do self/simple lymphatic drainage (SLD). I received holistic therapies which included aromatherapy and reiki as well as tremendous support. I was eventually discharged, since it was determined that I could take care of myself.

My daily routines include SLD, skincare, hydration, deep breathing, activity, and a healthy lifestyle to manage my lymphoedema. These tasks are an essential part of my daily routine.

We are all unique and therefore given time we adapt to doing what's right for us. I found answers to managing and controlling my lymphoedema did not come out of a medical textbook, it came from learning about myself and learning from others who live with lymphoedema. What works for me will not work necessarily work for someone else.

At no time during my cancer treatment was I told that the radiotherapy, while killing off any remaining cancer cells, would cause another problem. There wasn't much understanding, or information available when I received my diagnosis in May 2011.

Like many patients in the UK, I was given a list of all the things I would not be able to do, and how I might get a serious infection if I didn't follow this list religiously. This list of myths has no scientific significance, yes, we need guidelines and yes, we need to take sensible precautions. We do have to be extremely watchful looking for signs of infection and mindful of any further swelling in our affected areas. These precautions must not be allowed to rule our lives.

The list of dos and don'ts destroyed my enthusiasm for gardening because it advised covering your arms and legs, wearing gloves, and wearing sturdy shoes in case you pricked yourself and cause an infection. I used to like to get my hands in the earth, the feel of the soil and then to watch from the early stages of planting as my hard work blossomed. Life would have been so much simpler and less frightening if only the advice given at the time had been to take reasonable safeguards.

I believe you can accomplish whatever you feel capable of. The initial list of dos and don'ts that I was provided was unhelpful and had a negative impact on my mental health.

I've never had cellulitis, unlike other individuals with lymphoedema, and as far as I know, no one seems to know why some people are predisposed to this serious infection while others are not. My mother always had skin that healed quickly. No matter how deep the cut, she never developed an infection, never needed to go to Accident and Emergency, and recovered quite rapidly. I like to think I have inherited her quick healing skin and, therefore, cuts and grazes I get tend to heal quickly and without too much trouble.

Does lymphoedema spread? On the L-W-O Community Support Group, this query is frequently asked. I have thought about this a lot since I first started to understand my lymphoedema and the question remains unanswered. Was I predisposed to the problem before developing breast lymphoedema? For a non-medical person like me, the solution is too complicated to provide. But in November 2021, I was told that I had severe lymphoedema that affected my lower torso and waist.

My personal theory is that disease was present prior to being diagnosed with breast lymphoedema. The lymphoedema in the locations listed may have been caused by or brought on by certain medical events in my life. While this is supposition on my part, the signs and symptoms of breast lymphoedema that I encounter are the same as those I experience in the waist and torso. If I was to put a time scale on this, then I would suggest from the mid-nineties I started to experience problems, however, I wouldn't have been aware of lymphoedema at the time.

Patient Advocate

After spending two years learning about my disease, I unintentionally realised that in the UK there was a need for greater support. At that time, there were a few small lymphoedema online support groups in the UK.

For me, the entire process has been a steep learning curve and a period of personal growth. From the early days of information gathering following my

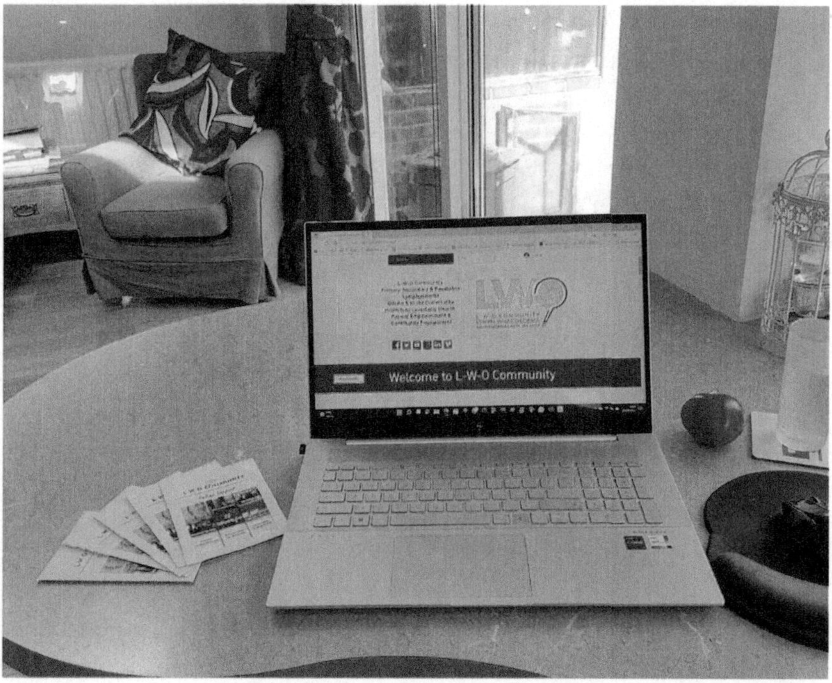

Gaynor Leech - LWO Community Home Office

diagnosis in 2011, to the 2013 launch of my initial lymphoedema website and Facebook social media page. This was soon followed by an online support group and other social media platforms. During that time, I was learning to live with lymphoedema and come to terms with what this meant for me and my life. When I first started, I had no plan, no background in social media, no knowledge of design, and no idea where this was heading. All I knew was that I wanted to make sure nobody else diagnosed with lymphoedema had the same feelings as I experienced.

Who would have imagined how my life would change in 2013, when I was 62 years old, and most people were approaching retirement. Did I ever imagine that L-W-O (lymph-what-oedema), which I founded out of irritation over the ignorance and, worse, disinformation surrounding lymphoedema, would develop and expand into the supportive community it is today? We have now transitioned from lymph-what-oedema to L-W-O Community. It has undoubtedly been an emotional rollercoaster, with feelings of rage, frustration, rejection, sadness, exhaustion, intense joy, thankfulness, and a sense of accomplishment.

I initially encountered a lot of opposition from medical professionals when I suggested starting an online support group. Breaking through the barriers and opposition of those who found it difficult to adopt online support groups is truly significant for the lymphoedema community.

However, people living with lymphoedema embraced us with open arms right from the beginning. I was happy that 37 people had joined our support group in our first month, to the community we are today, which numbers over 4,500 people.

Digital health and technology-enabled care are not new ideas, and I fully realise that they exclude many people given the difficult financial conditions we are in currently. However, it is crucial to provide our members and the larger patient community with the resources for self-care through our online communities, today more than ever.

Much to my surprise, we are growing a strong UK base that has gone well beyond our borders, giving the L-W-O Community a voice and a global audience. Online communities are prospering, and patient empowerment has grown significantly, whether you are a member of a lymphoedema community or another group that supports or shares your health interests.

Now, wherever you may be in the world, people who have lymphoedema have organised themselves to help one another. Together, we can provide support 365/6 days a year, around-the-clock. Our online platforms allow people to express themselves, and we never pass judgement. When there is no other help available, we offer a valuable listening service.

Many of us believe the health system, which includes diagnosis, treatment recommendations, and support, has failed us. Unfortunately, some lymphoedema patients do not receive the care or services from the NHS or their local health service, and there is a lack of understanding of our needs. This is likely to be because most clinicians receive very little training on lymphoedema and the lymphatic system, therefore, do not understand how our immune systems are linked. A greater understanding is needed, how lymphatic health is important to our overall health.

Our community values patient empowerment, and by realising that every one of us has a role to play, we can work together to achieve our shared objectives of increasing awareness about lymphoedema and promoting lymphatic health.

Everything I write or design is based on mine and our members experience. Our goal is to arm individuals with the skills to speak up for themselves, particularly when dealing with clinician resistance. This empowers our members to become their own advocates and make well-informed decisions.

We do this successfully through our online posters, presentations, social media, and website. Not only do we provide support, information, and signposting, but we encourage our members to talk about living with lymphoedema. I am convinced that interaction amongst our members has decreased self-isolation and improved their mental health.

I recognise that everyone of us is fiercely protective of the unique groups or organisations we build, but this is the time to work together. For those of us with lymphoedema, community involvement is crucial and one of the most effective instruments for amplifying our voice.

In the beginning, I could never have envisioned being requested to collaborate with other lymphoedema organisations like the British Lymphology Society, European Patient Advocacy group, or International Lymphoedema Framework. Neither could I have dreamt that I would write book chapters or articles to be published or co-present workshops.

In September 2023, L-W-O Community will celebrate its 10th anniversary. My message then and now is ***"Lymphoedema exists, we exist".***

TOP TIP!

Learn to understand yourself and what works for you.

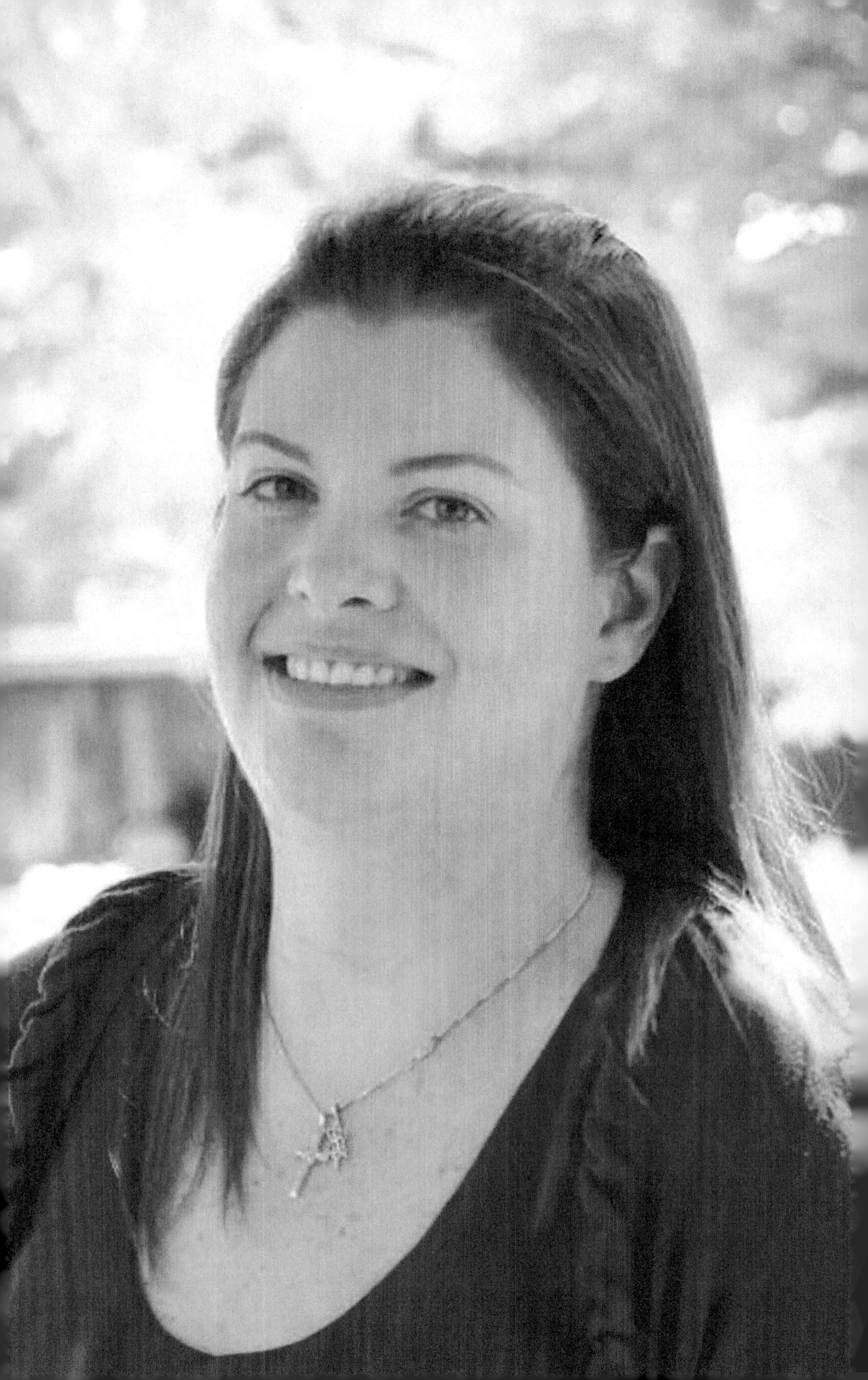

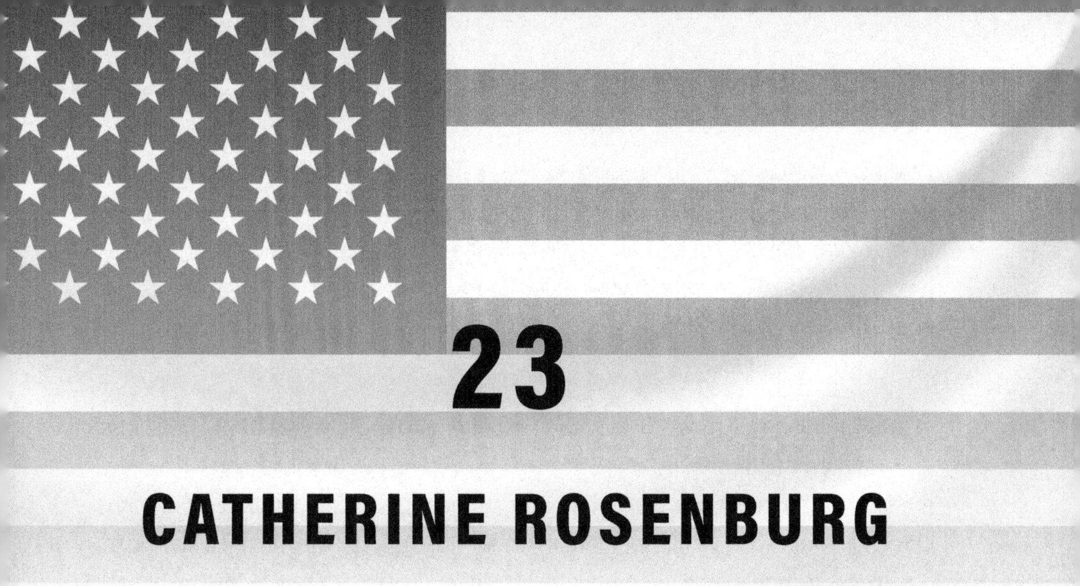

23

CATHERINE ROSENBURG

> ***The entire process of my medical journey has been unpredictable and has traversed various challenging areas.***

As a young child, I was diagnosed with a rare form of cancer known as Synovial Cell Sarcoma. It was a shocking diagnosis, especially for someone my age. At just eight years old, I underwent a surgical resection of the tumor followed by intense radiation treatment. However, after completing the radiation therapy, I noticed that my left leg remained swollen and larger than my right leg. It was a constant reminder of the battle I had fought.

I returned to my pediatric Radiation Oncologist at The Hospital of the University of Pennsylvania, where I received the official diagnosis of left lower extremity lymphedema. Unfortunately, there were no local specialists treating pediatric lymphedema patients, so my lymphedema remained untreated for over 15 years. That was until one day when I saw a television commercial about a doctor who treated lymphedema using compression wraps and lymphatic drainage.

Feeling hopeful and with nothing to lose, I decided to call the number on the advertisement. To my surprise, the doctor was located less than an hour away from my residence. I began undergoing Manual Lymphatic Drainage and compression therapy five days a week. I was determined to learn as much as I could about my condition and took it upon myself to become proficient in compression wrapping techniques.

In 2005, my journey took a turn when I experienced my first battle with cellulitis. This marked the beginning of a series of severe and intense infections. I sought the help of an infectious disease doctor to manage these constant infections. Over the course of a year, I spent more time in the hospital than in my own house due to the severity of the infections. In 2014, after about 30 bouts of MRSA-based cellulitis, flesh-eating pseudomonas, and Vancomycin-Resistant Enterococcus (VRE), I was diagnosed as a carrier of MRSA.

In the same year, I faced another challenge when it was determined that my left hip needed to be replaced. The pain, discomfort, and weakness were unbearable. Despite the complexity of the surgery due to my lymphedema and the need for a six-hour procedure, I successfully underwent hip replacement surgery performed by a renowned orthopedic oncologist. I was relieved to have my hip replaced, and everything seemed to be going well. I returned to work as an elementary special education teacher, only to discover that something wasn't right with my hip replacement. I reached out to my orthopedic oncologist, and upon examination, my hip dislocated out the front, an uncommon occurrence. The orthopedic team attempted a closed reduction but unfortunately failed.

As a result, I underwent another surgery to replace the liner on my hip. Before changing anything, the surgeon surgically put my hip back in place and let my leg hang off the operating room table. Unfortunately, my hip dislocated again within seconds, leading to the first-ever diagnosis of lymphedema-associated hip dislocation at Jefferson Hospital. To prevent further dislocations, my hip replacement liner was changed to a constrained liner.

In 2014, I reached a point where I was determined to take control of my medical condition and find the most effective treatments. My continuous infections and lack of improvement led me to research surgical interventions for lymphedema. In 2015, I opted for a vascularized lymph node transplant from the supraclavicular to the groin region. Initially, the procedure seemed successful, but over time, it became evident that it was causing further issues with my lymphatic system and hip replacement.

My medical providers began calling me a medical mystery as my body seemed to defy expectations. In 2016, my left hip internally rotated, and no one could determine the cause. Extensive imaging studies were conducted, but nothing conclusive was found. My orthopedic oncologist recommended that I look further into getting my lymphedema under control with the hopes that it would help improve the status of my hip replacement.

In February 2018, I flew down to Dallas, Texas to see Dr. Alexander Nguyen from the Integrative Lymphedema Institute at Medical City Dallas Hospital. During my consultation with Dr. Nguyen, I learned that my condition was much worse than anyone had expected, and I needed further medical treatment. Dr. Nguyen scheduled surgery for me in May 2018. My mom, who has been my biggest support, accompanied me to Dallas, and we had a final pre-operative appointment with Dr. Nguyen. However, during that appointment, Dr. Nguyen realized that his initial plan needed to be revised due to the increased fibrosis found in my left groin. He recommended additional imaging to plan the best surgical outcome for me. Once the revised plan was in place, Dr. Nguyen proceeded with my surgery as planned.

The entire process of my medical journey has been unpredictable and has traversed various challenging areas. During my vascularized lymph node transplant surgery using my omentum, Dr. Nguyen discovered a radiation tissue growth that had started to grow from a previous vascularized lymph node transfer, posing a significant risk near my femoral artery. Luckily, Dr. Nguyen was able to address it during the surgery, and my leg was no longer internally rotated. The surgery was long and meticulous, but it was ultimately a huge success. After a lengthy recovery, I was able to return to work, knowing that there was still a part two of the treatment to come. To facilitate proper reconnection, Dr. Nguyen intentionally caused a hernia, which could only be repaired 11 months after the lymphatic surgery once lymphangiogenesis occurred in the groin region.

Back in New Jersey, I resumed working full-time while also undergoing Complete Decongestive Therapy three times a week. Over time, my leg started to improve, but I had to constantly modify my compression needs based on how I was feeling on a particular day. However, out of the blue, things quickly reversed, and I couldn't understand why.

Then, on August 5, 2021, I had the opportunity to meet with Dr. Jasmine Zheng, a specialist in lymphedema at The Hospital of the University of Pennsylvania. I felt relieved to finally have a doctor who understood lymphedema and could help me during challenging times, even though I didn't anticipate any difficulties in the near future. Unfortunately, in August 2021, I began experiencing increased abdominal swelling despite my compression regimen. I started tracking various factors like diet, exercise, and circumferential measurements to identify any patterns, but everything seemed random. By the end of September 2021, I had gained 37 pounds in just 30 days, without making any changes to my lifestyle or compression routine.

Concerned about my symptoms, I reached out to my primary care physician for insights. We ran standard bloodwork and hormone panels, which initially showed normal results. However, the hormone levels raised red flags, considering I had a hysterectomy and only one remaining ovary. My estrogen levels were significantly higher than expected. I consulted my gynecologist, who conducted further testing, confirming the abnormal estrogen levels. Although it wasn't clear how it related to my lymphatic dysfunction, my gynecologist suspected a connection due to my medical history.

In November 2021, I contacted Dr. Zheng again and informed her of the developments since my last visit in August. She ordered a STAT CT scan of my abdomen and pelvis, which didn't reveal anything alarming. However, I persisted in requesting an evaluation of my central lymphatics, as I could sense that my lymphatic system was involved somehow.

Dr. Zheng referred me to Dr. Maxim Itkin, an interventional radiologist specializing in imaging of the central lymphatic system at the Hospital of the University of Pennsylvania, for an evaluation of my central lymphatic system.

In February 2022, I underwent a Dynamic Contrast MR – Lymphangiogram, which revealed that my thoracic duct was torturous at the distal end. This indicated that my lymphatic system was not functioning properly, and the twisted and obstructed thoracic duct, responsible for draining lymph from the lower half of my body, required attention. As a result, I returned for an angioplasty attempt on my left thoracic duct, accompanied by a live lymphangiogram under anesthesia. During the procedure, Dr. Itkin determined that angioplasty alone would not be sufficient to fix my thoracic duct and recommended a lymphovenous anastomosis. This complex procedure involved the collaboration of Dr. Itkin, the interventional radiologist, and Dr. Stephen Kovach, a plastic surgeon.

At that time, I was aware of the waiting period required for this procedure due to the need to coordinate the schedules of two surgeons and secure a specific hybrid operating room. Although I was hoping to finish the school year before undergoing surgery, my symptoms began to worsen, and I advocated for an earlier date. Unfortunately, due to the complexity of the procedure and scheduling constraints, it was not possible to expedite the surgery.

Consequently, I had to miss the end of the school year as I struggled with prolonged periods of difficulty in speaking due to reduced oxygen levels caused by fluid retention in my chest. My oxygen saturation levels dropped into the 80s each night, and I experienced extreme fatigue and weakness due to severely low iron saturation levels. The abdominal swelling, pain, and uncontrollable weight gain added to my distress. Nightly fluctuations of approximately 17 pounds of fluid occurred despite no changes in my diet or exercise routine.

Finally, the day of my surgery, July 18th, had arrived. I was filled with hope and anticipation, ready for things to improve. Both Dr. Itkin and Dr. Kovach visited me in the pre-surgery holding area, where they graciously addressed any last-minute questions my mom and I had. Dr. Kovach explained that if Dr. Itkin encountered difficulties accessing my thoracic duct, the surgery would have to be aborted as he wouldn't be able to proceed. Thankfully, Dr. Itkin's determination during the procedure was unwavering. Despite facing challenges in identifying my thoracic duct, he persisted and never gave up. Eventually, the duct was successfully located, leading to a tremendous breakthrough.

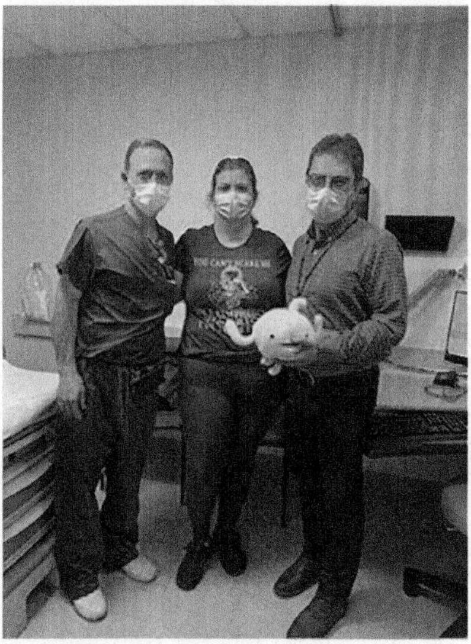

Dr Kovach, Catherine Rosenberg and Dr Itkin

Since July 2022, I have been steadily improving each month. Significant progress was observed within the first four weeks following the procedure, and even now,

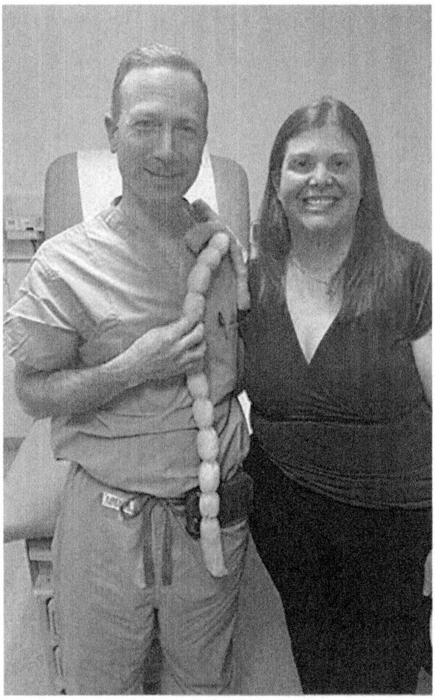

Dr Kovach and Catherine Rosenberg

at eight months post-surgery, I continue to experience positive advancements. Among the notable improvements are the resolution of SVTs (supraventricular tachycardias) originating from my heart, the regulation of both my iron saturation and estrogen levels, and the freedom from wearing abdominal compression garments due to the successful repair of my thoracic duct.

Although the road to recovery was long and challenging, I persevered. With the unwavering support of my medical team and the love of my dear ones, I managed to overcome the complexities associated with my central lymphatic dysfunction. Now, I am living a joyous and healthy life, free from the debilitating symptoms that once plagued me.

Managing lymphedema can be a trial-and-error process, and it's essential to advocate for yourself and seek professionals who are willing to help you find answers. If you feel that your current management strategies are no longer effective, don't hesitate to explore other options and seek guidance. Remember, even if symptoms may not seem directly related to the lymphatic system, they could still be connected.

TOP TIP!

Managing lymphedema can be a trial-and-error process. Trust your instincts and keep searching for the right solutions to improve your well-being.

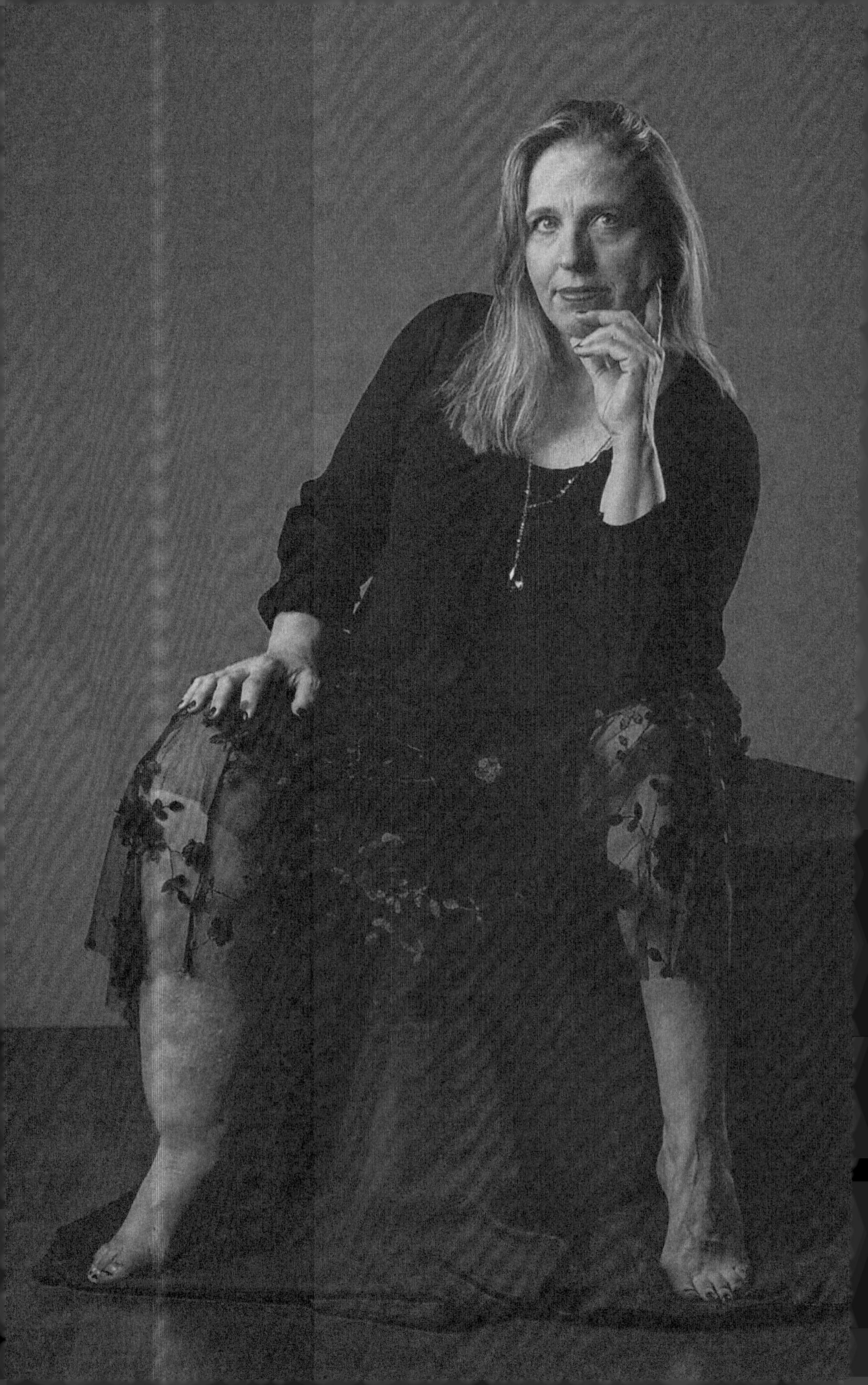

24

VALERIA AMIZICH

> ***The key lies in educating ourselves about the affected body part, viewing it as an infinite mountain to climb each day without ever giving up.***

I am Valeria Amizich, known as @valeria_amizich, and I am 55 years old. I reside in Sitges, Barcelona, Spain and work as a nursing assistant at Hospital Sant Antoni Abad Consorci Sanitari de Alt Penedès Garraf. Since I was 15 years old, I have been living with primary lymphedema in my right extremity. Lymphedema is a condition caused by lymphatic dysfunction, resulting in the accumulation of protein-rich fluid in the interstitial space. This leads to swelling or enlargement of the affected body region. In my case, I was born with a lack of lymphatic ducts and lymph node hypoplasia in my leg.

Lymphedema is a chronic, progressive, and disabling disease that requires constant, often intensive, and complex care. Each person's experience with lymphedema is unique, necessitating personalized evaluations, treatments, and techniques. Physiotherapists play an irreplaceable and indispensable role in providing constant support and guidance until the patient gains autonomy. While professional lymphotherapists are essential, patients themselves and their relatives can also contribute significantly to maintaining and achieving favorable results.

It is crucial to strive for autonomy in managing lymphedema, as the treatment is complex. This involves understanding self-drainage techniques, incorporating diaphragmatic breathing, engaging in myolymphokinetic exercises, practicing stretching, and utilizing multi-component multilayer compression bandages, gloves, and custom-made compression stockings. The journey has not been easy, and I have gone through various emotional processes, including anger, helplessness, despair, anguish, sadness, joy, euphoria, and frustration.

My search for a diagnosis and treatment lasted 14 years, during which I faced numerous infections and hospitalizations. Eventually, a compassionate healthcare professional shed light on my condition and introduced a complex decongestant treatment, requiring patience, perseverance, and determination. I have educated myself on the physiology and anatomy of the lymphatic system, learning to respect pressure, relaxation, direction, and rhythm when performing manual lymphatic drainage (MLD). With my hands and visualization techniques, I have created pathways for lymphatic flow, effectively draining toxins from my leg.

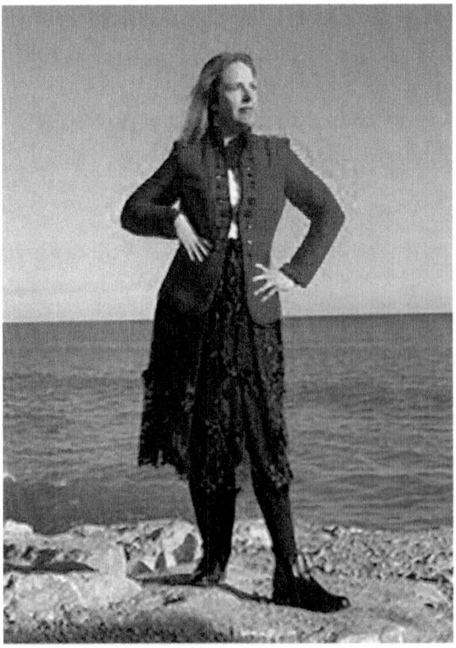

Valeria Amizich - You possess great strength. Never give up!

Bandaging my leg became a daily ritual, repeating it week after week, month after month, until today. In late 2019, I was diagnosed with Grade 4 breast carcinoma in Situ, and underwent surgery, followed by 25 sessions of radiotherapy, all while navigating the challenges posed by the Covid-19 pandemic. I have overcome this as well. The key lies in educating ourselves about the affected body part, viewing it as an infinite mountain to climb each day without ever giving up.

Though our stories, countries, ages, and treatment paths may differ, we are united as a great family through our shared experiences. Together with organizations like Limfacall and others, we stand strong. Lymphedema is always in motion, cyclic like life itself, with its ups and downs. Remember, you are not alone; don't lose momentum. I extend my hand to embrace and support you because I, too, am affected by this condition.

Just as we need air to breathe and water to live, we also require our hands to drain toxins and experience relief in the affected area. Resilience is a constant presence in our lives. Engage in activities that bring you joy, seek emotional and therapeutic support from family and friends. Everything is possible as long as you believe in it. You possess great strength, and you are continually learning. Never give up.

TOP TIP!

Attitude is EVERYTHING

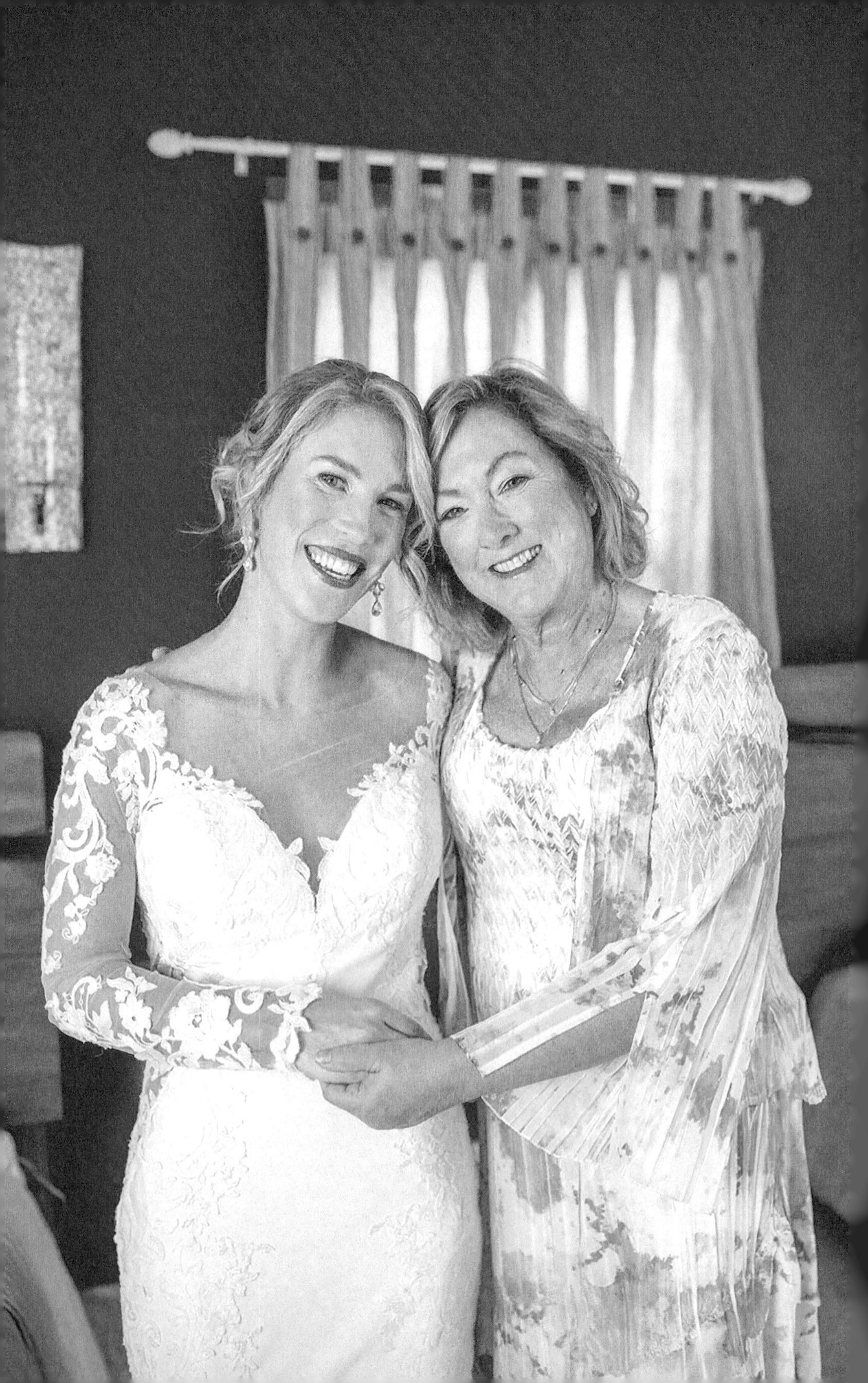

25

TINA & BABZ JACKSON

> ***I would recommend to anyone who is newly diagnosed to seek immediate help once the swelling starts.***

I was diagnosed with stage two Breast Cancer (triple negative) in December 2006. I underwent a bilateral mastectomy (both breasts removed) in January of 2007. Then followed by chemotherapy and radiation that winter throughout the summer.

Shortly after that I developed lymphedema. It was moderate for a while and I was referred to physical therapy and fitted for a compression sleeve, but I only wore it when I flew.

I must admit, I wasn't the most compliant patient. I was frustrated and really hated wrapping my arm, especially in the summer, as it was too hot. Then things got worse and I got cellulitis twice in a year and a half, which I think woke me up to the seriousness of this diagnosis. It was a very uneasy feeling not to be able to help myself or understand why I developed it.

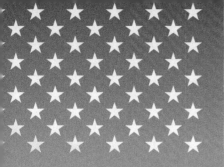

I remember when the swelling finally affected my hand which blew up. I was so bummed I couldn't even wear my wedding bands. My sister Dee recommended I switch them to my right hand. That made me feel a little better but I was so angry I couldn't get the swelling down. There were shirts I couldn't wear, and I felt in constant discomfort. It was very upsetting. It was affecting my daily life.

I would recommend to anyone who is newly diagnosed to seek immediate help once the swelling starts. I would recommend talking to your doctor right away and being referred to a certified lymphedema therapist. The intensive education and therapy really gets the swelling down and under control and teaches you how to be able to manage yourself. My daughter and I want to share our story so that it can help someone who is in a similar situation. That's where my daughter Babz comes in.

My daughter is an occupational therapist and a certified lymphedema therapist through the Klose Lymphedema Therapist Certification course. When she returned home from completing the course she got right to work on my arm. The course provided her with the knowledge, confidence and skills to help me get my lymphedema under control.

She treated my arm when it was truly at its worst point. She was determined and helped me to help myself.

Above all, finally I was given the tools to help myself. Learning how to self-massage and move the fluid myself was amazing. Everyone should know how to do this if they are struggling with lymphedema like I was. Also, I've been doing lymphatic flow yoga with Babz for over two years. Yoga with Babz has also been an addition to my success story. And yoga was never something I even thought could help, or that I thought I could do! I hope my story will help someone to get educated and find a therapist like Babz who's dedicated to helping us get our lymphedema under control and managed and get back to our best self!!! I call it my new normal!!

Babz not only treated my lymphedema, but she helped me with my whole body's health. She asked about my diet, my water consumption, my exercise and most importantly she taught me how to do self-lymphatic drainage. She had me fitted for new daytime compression garments as well as a night compression garment. I lost weight; I drink a lot more water during the day and I looked at all aspects of my life to see where I could be healthier. It was a lot but so worth it!! I could see the fluid leaving my arm and the swelling reduced greatly. And the lymphedema has stayed down. I now understand what I am doing, and why I am doing it. Today my arm is under control, and I am managing my lymphedema through the many ways listed above, and now lymphatic flow yoga is in my weekly routine.

Hi, I'm Babz, Tina's daughter.

When I heard about the lymphedema training I knew I had to do it. I watched my mom battle breast cancer, and struggle with lymphedema and I needed to help her. I came home from the intensive hands-on training and got right into it.

With the completion of the Klose training, I finally understood what the lymphatic system was, why my mom had developed lymphedema from having breast cancer, and most importantly the tools to help someone successfully manage living with lymphedema.

I have watched my mom improve her lymphedema significantly and most importantly her wellbeing. Her knowledge of her own body continues to grow and I am so excited to continue to help individuals like my mom. If you or someone you know has lymphedema, please share this with them.

Below are many of the ways that my mom and I have found helps to decrease swelling, improve range of motion and improve quality of life while living with lymphedema.

1. **Daily Self- Manual Lymphatic Drainage**
   (Through hand massage and/or dry brushing). Understanding the pathways that the lymph fluid moves is critical to improving lymphatic drainage of your affected area.

2. **Exercise**
   Rebounding, lymphatic flow yoga, aquatic therapy, functional mobility (walking), and resistive exercise. Improving muscular strength and activating the muscle pumps in the body helps to increase lymph drainage.

3. **Compression Bandaging & Fitting for Compression Garments**
   We started with a strict two-week compression bandaging protocol and then trial and error with multiple day and night sleeves, gloves, gauntlets. We just kept on trying until we found a great routine!

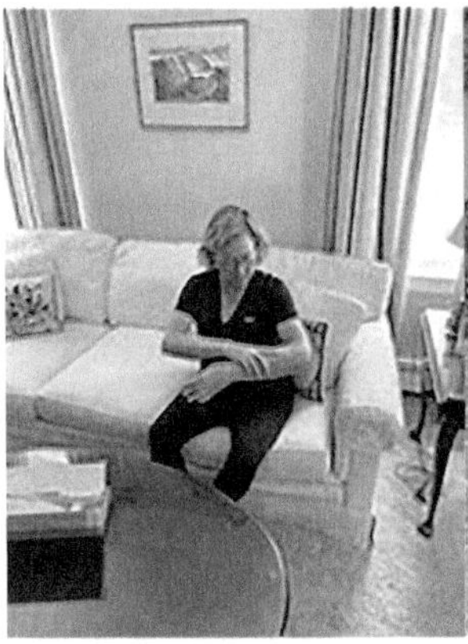
Tina Jackson - Self-MLD

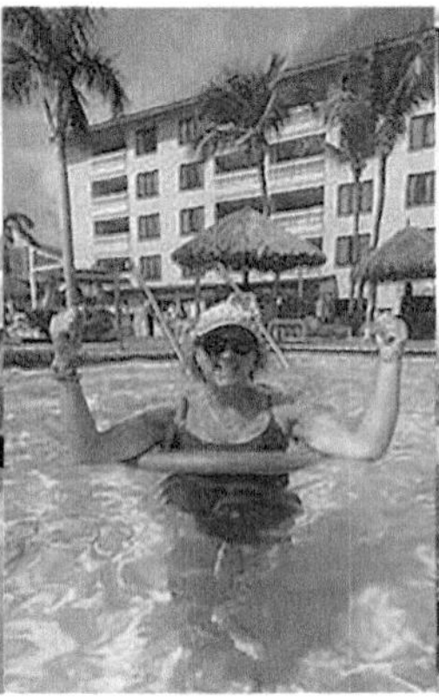
Tina Jackson - Exercise

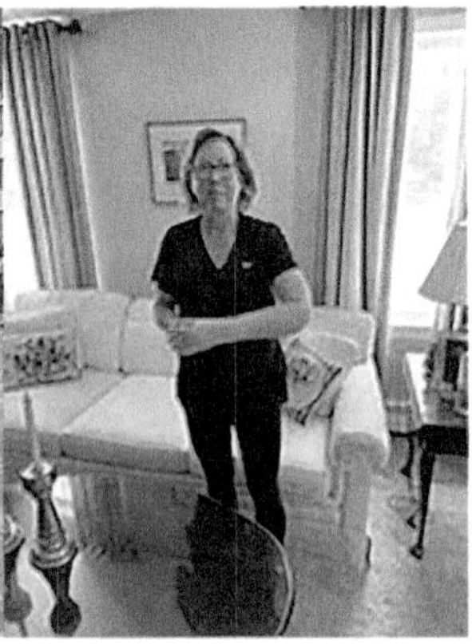
Tina Jackson - Arm Compression

4 **Daily Routine**
Checking in with daily routines to promote lymphatic system health; nutrition, self-care, skin hygiene, weight loss (maintain a recommended body mass index).

If you have lymphedema, lipedema, or are at risk or have a lymphatic disorder please reach out to me! My hope is that my free education and resources on my website *https://www.balancewithbabz.com/* and YouTube channel *https://www.youtube.com/@balancewithbabz* and my lymphatic flow yoga programs will continue to help people like my mom. Together we are stronger.

TOP TIP!

Through Babz teaching me lymphatic flow yoga, I have learned a self-manual lymph drainage routine that I do daily. The self MLD routine combined with the yoga stretches has helped me to stay active, and to increase my balance.

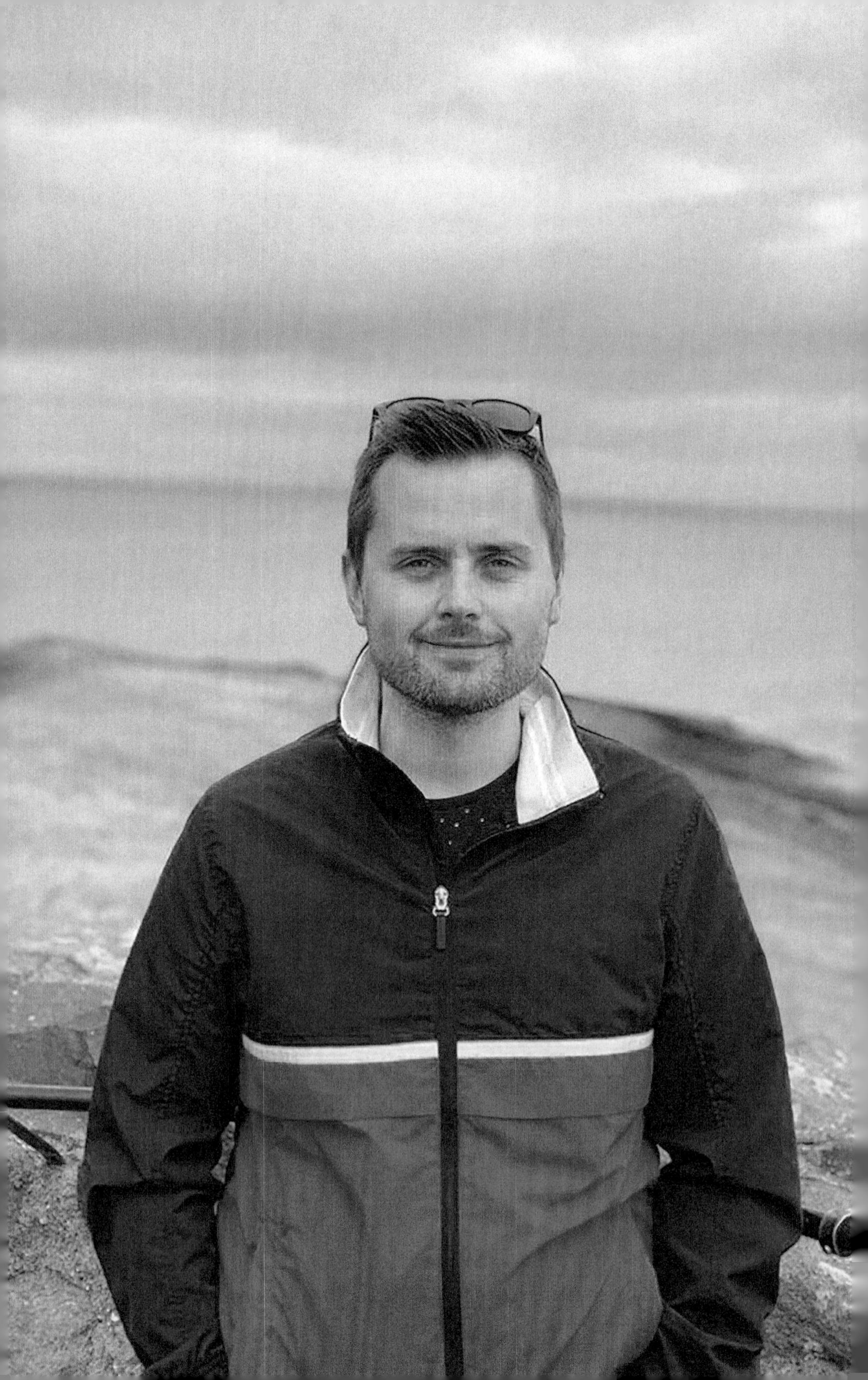

26

TOM NEILSON

> ***We have to remember that if well managed, lymphoedema shouldn't be stopping you from living normal day to day life.***

My name is Tom Neilson, and at the time of writing this, I am 36 and live in the UK. I have been living with lymphoedema in my left leg since April 2019.

From what I have learnt during my time living with this condition, I fall into a rare category. Firstly, being a young man and secondly having primary lymphoedema. Like many other people, I had never heard of lymphoedema and never thought living with a chronic condition was something I was going to have to deal with, certainly not in my thirties. The first signs came out of nowhere, in my case, at work one afternoon. I remember it quite vividly, just noticing my lower left leg had swelled up. I was perplexed more than anything, little did I know how much my life was going to change. I arranged an appointment at the doctor's the very same afternoon. They were concerned it could be a Deep Vein Thrombosis. Early symptoms of lymphoedema present much like many other conditions. I was directed to A&E as a result, where after many hours of nervously waiting, including for the results of a blood test, it was determined there was no blood clot.

So, I left the hospital with some blood thinner injections as a precaution but still no closer to finding out what was happening. I am almost certain anyone with lymphoedema can probably sympathise with this situation, certainly in the earlier days, when you had no idea where to turn and were frantically searching the internet for any ideas about why your body was doing this.

In the weeks and months after my first GP visit, I made many return trips, but got no closer to a diagnosis. Sometimes it felt like things were improving but then it would get worse again. Looking back, I get incredibly frustrated because I now see how vital these earlier days would have been to seriously get on top of what was happening and be able to slow down the progress of my leg swelling.

I was referred for investigative blood tests, X-rays and ultrasounds. In the end, after doing my own further research, I had my suspicions my problem was lymphoedema. It soon became apparent that lymphoedema is a not a well-known and often misunderstood condition, even amongst those in the medical profession. So, at my next appointment, armed with all the knowledge I had learnt, I asked my GP for some compression garments and a 12-week referral to a vascular specialist. They agreed and I finally thought I was getting somewhere!

During this time, I was trying to adjust to what I was learning and wearing these compression garments daily. I had no doubt they were helping me physically, but mentally they were really making me feel miserable but at least I was making some progress. It was around early September 2019 that I had my first experience with cellulitis. I was on a small break with my partner at the time and we had done a lot of walking on this day, I remember that evening lying in bed and my left thigh was in so much pain, quite red and inflamed and I could barely walk.

A trip to the hospital later and being sent away with some antibiotics meant I was soon on the mend, but it really did make me think about how this was not just a simple swelling and if not monitored correctly, could develop into something more serious.

Over the years, I've not had such a bad repeat of that evening, but this only comes with the knowledge of what I have learnt and being vigilant about such things. It also gave me a new thing to be discussing with vascular specialist at my upcoming appointment. However, I was going to be let down again. Just two weeks before I received a letter to inform me it had been cancelled and rescheduled for another 12 weeks' time.

I was feeling broken at this point; I was now eight months into this spiral with no confirmed diagnosis and felt I had no choice but to have a private consultation. As ever, money makes things happen and after spending £180, a BUPA consultant saw me the following week. He determined I had no issues with my vein flow and was certain it was lymphoedema but asked for an MRI to rule out anything "sinister". Fortunately, this came back all clear and he was able to link up my results for the newly rescheduled appointment.

I was finally able to meet an NHS lymphoedema consultant just before Covid-19 turned the world upside down. It was such a relief to meet someone who understood my condition, I was able to ask as many questions as I wanted and was measured for full leg compression garments. Looking back though, it was interesting to just be told you have lymphoedema in the same way you might have the flu or something else trivial, not learning this was the start of a lifelong change for me.

I left with what felt a degree of closure confirming what I had been researching had been proved correct and that I was on the right path. At the follow up appointment, I could see the progress the compression had made with improved measurements.

We also discussed the potential of funding being made available to do a course in DLT (Decongestive Lymphatic Therapy). I jumped at the chance to do this and in February 2021, I finally met Dawn Heal, a lymphoedema nurse specialist at the Candover Clinic in Basingstoke. Dawn explained that the DLT process involves three weeks of leg bandaging with nine MLD (Manual Lymphatic Drainage) sessions. I was really happy with the leg improvement from this over the two treatments periods I had with Dawn who has years of lymphoedema experience and is deeply passionate and knowledgeable. I feel extremely fortunate to have been referred to her for this treatment.

I have appointments every six months at the same hospital, with my nurse, Amy Hinsley, who is also knowledgeable about this condition. We re-measure my leg to order new garments, wraps and whatever else is needed. It is great to be under such a caring department as I know what a postcode lottery it can be for some fellow sufferers to get the treatment they need.

Lymphoedema has meant I've had to make such a huge adjustment to my life. I never thought as a man in his early thirties, this would be a condition I would have to deal with. I've found that having the support to help you power on through is particularly important. If I look back over the last few years, there is no denying it has been a struggle at times, both mentally and physically draining, there is no decision I make now without thinking how it will affect my "lymphie leg".

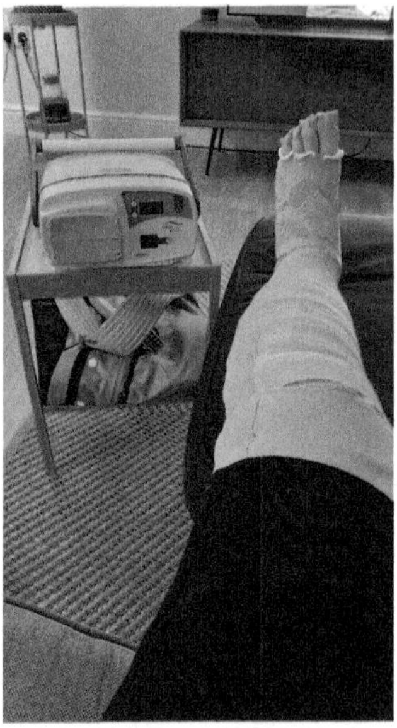

Tom Neilson - Self-care with elevation, wraps and Compression Pump

It is on my mind an awful lot of the day, usually when adjusting my compression garments! Not to mention the various other aspects of my life that have changed, including frequent prescription requests, visits to the hospital, keeping an eye on subtle changes and being vigilant for my next bout of cellulitis. I am truly fortunate to have my fiancé, who has been my rock throughout this process, and I would not be as strong as I am without him.

One of the hardest things to deal with when living with Lymphoedema is being disciplined with the necessary routines, especially with regards to self-care. This is my top tip when learning how to live with it as best you can. We all know what works best for us as individuals, I personally have a compression pump which I purchased after completing my sessions with Dawn. I use this daily, and it really does help with recreating the MLD sessions you would have in a clinical setting. Also, keeping my affected limb raised, skin care, and diet all play a part in keeping on top of this condition and stopping it from making more progress.

The most important thing to remember here is this is a chronic condition. I have now been living with it for over 4 years, I have learnt a lot in this time, and it's important to remember, we are only human. Of course, I have days where I am not as disciplined as I should be in using my pump, or I wanted some unhealthy food etc. It is easy to feel overwhelmed, but you can only do your best to live with it.

It's also important to simply carry on with your life! We have to remember that if well managed, lymphoedema shouldn't be stopping you from living normal day to day life. I'm a Heavy Goods Vehicle driver for a supermarket so I'm quite active day to day. My fiancé' and I have regular holidays in the UK, with one our favourite activities being exploring castles and cathedrals, which can give you quite a high step count after a long day! Since having my condition, we've even climbed up Cheddar Gorge. I never let my condition stop me from doing anything.

I have also found support from multiple sources online. I co-own and administrate a Facebook group called "Lymphoedema Sufferers UK." I frequently post to get involved with the community offering positivity, advice, guidance, and support. We have now grown to over three thousand members and it continues to grow every day.

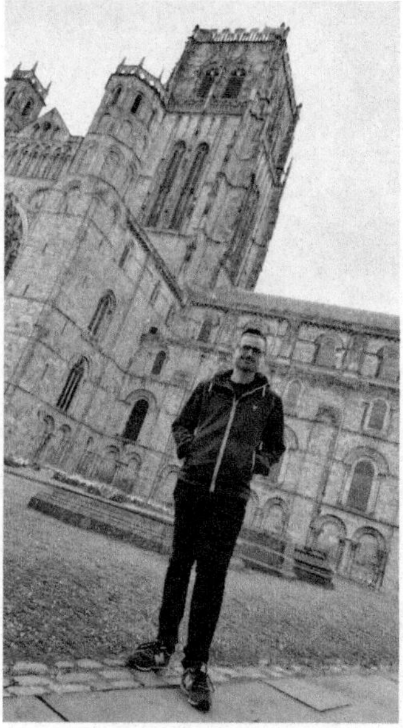

Tom Neilson - Not letting lymphoedema rule his life.

I'm also in regular contact with other members of various UK lymphoedema groups and the founder of Lymphoedema United, Matt Hazledine. We have regular catch ups with ideas about how best to bring our community together.

I look to the future with a sense of optimism, this journey so far has taught me an awful lot about my resilience and embracing this new part of my life. For most of us, lymphoedema is a chronic condition that will require constant attention and adjustment. There will be bad days, but the key is our positive attitude.

TOP TIP!

One of the hardest things to deal with when living with Lymphoedema is being disciplined with the necessary routines, especially with regards to self-care. Find out what works for you and stick with it!

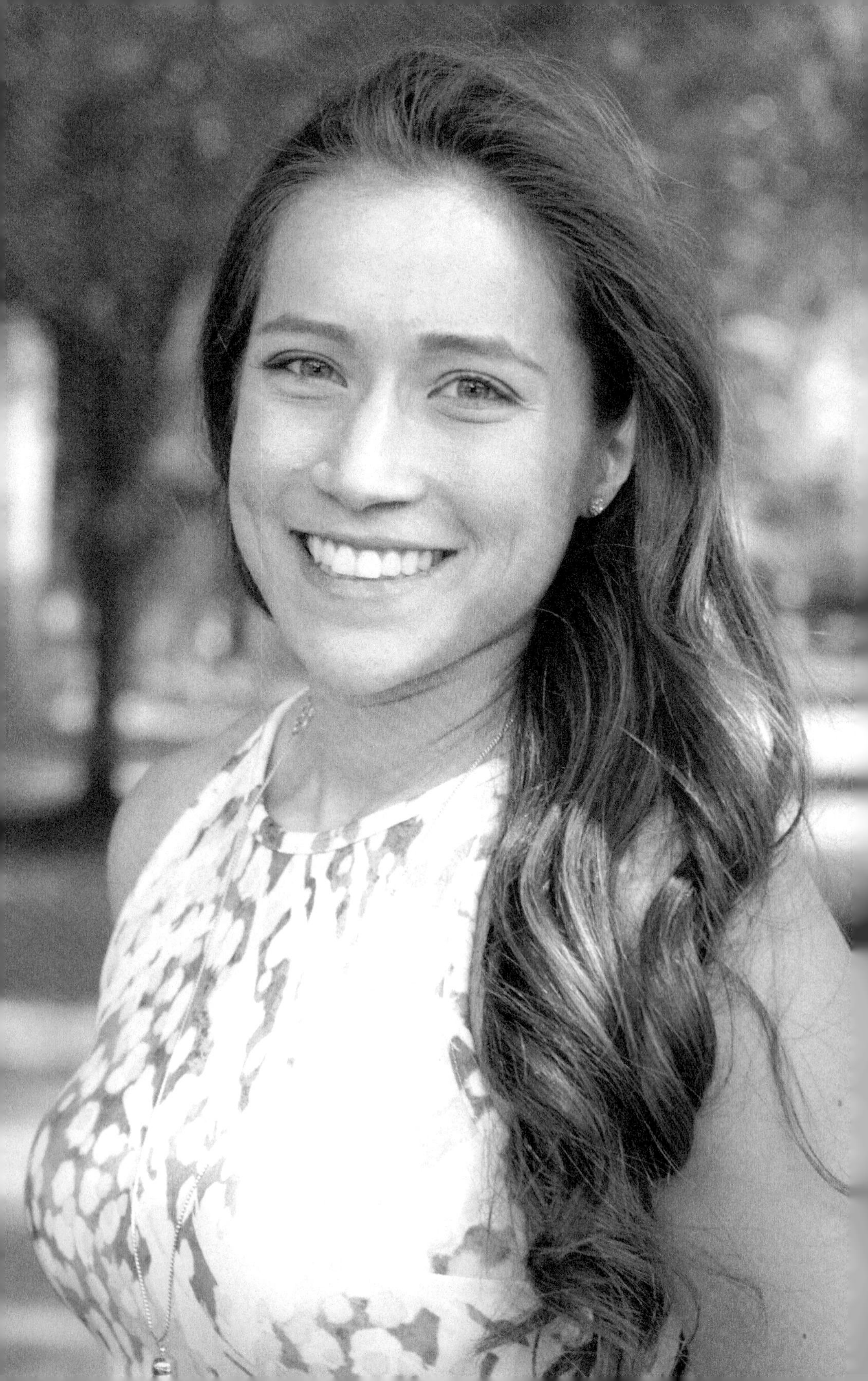

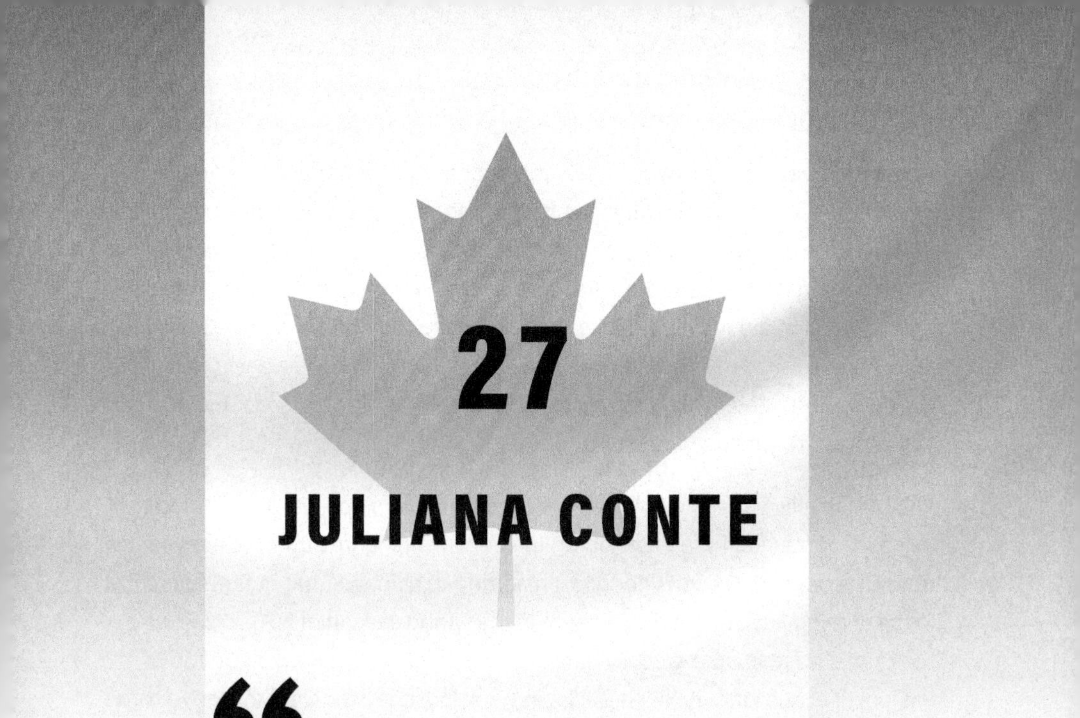

27

JULIANA CONTE

> ***There are people who are suffering from the mental, emotional, and physical effects of Lymphedema, and I want to help them get through things that I didn't think I was going to get through.***

The most obvious thing that sucks about lymphedema is the constant swelling and never-ending treatments. Living with lymphedema is like sitting in a rowboat with a hole in the bottom and trying to stay afloat by scooping the water out with a cup. If you stop scooping, even just to take a break, you will have a bigger problem on your hands, and if you give up entirely, you will sink. This condition can be relentless, progressive, and exhausting. When my swelling began 12 years ago, I was so focused on keeping myself from sinking physically that I overlooked the detrimental effects that lymphedema was having on every other facet of my life. Today, my goal is to help other lymphedema patients recognize and care for their emotional, mental, and spiritual needs, just as much as their physical ones.

I could tell you a story about how my "successful" hyper-productive life was brought to a screeching halt by the abrupt onset of a chronic disease – a disease that would strip me of my joy, confidence, and hope. I could tell you about how lymphedema left me deformed and how it distorted my perception of the world and how I fit in it. I felt disqualified before I ever really had a chance to run the race. I had worked my butt off since the age of 4, training every day and playing multiple sports determined to pay for school with an athletic scholarship. I had to learn self-discipline to power through tough times.

In 2010, I finally made it to college on a soccer scholarship and I just wanted to fit in. I had a great freshman season on the field, winning freshman of the year for my conference. I was considering transferring to a school that better suited me in the coming year, but during a game in the spring season of 2011, a player from the opposing team came down hard with the heel of her cleat on the top of my left foot. It hurt a lot, but I don't like losing, so I loosened my cleat to relieve some of the pressure from the swelling, and I kept playing. By the time I was ready to go to bed that night, the swelling had spread up my leg and my lower leg had become an unhealthy blue color. It wasn't for a few days that my trainers paid attention to how bad my leg looked and took me to the ER where they searched intensively for blood clots but never found any. There were only a few weeks left in the semester and by the time summer break came I had been diagnosed with lymphedema and May Thurner syndrome. My left iliac vein was 90% collapsed, resulting in severely restricted blood flow in my left leg, explaining the painfully swollen blue leg. Yet I was told to go home and "try to enjoy my family and have a normal summer." I don't remember much about that summer, other than I didn't enjoy much of anything. Every step I took was excruciating and, in my mind, my body was deformed and ugly.

For years, I felt like I was sinking and nothing could distract me from the misery of my reality. I was ridiculed about my leg. I felt dismissed and misunderstood by almost everyone. But over the years my pain has refined me in a way that I believe is only possible through struggle. I have learned things and grown in ways that have led me to where I am now, and I've never been this deeply happy and at peace with myself and my life. I feel like I'm finally becoming the person I was meant to be. And when I think about why it took me so long to get here, I realize I was always resisting. In times when it felt like life wasn't going my way, I put my head down and worked harder to get whatever it was that I thought I wanted. You might think that after my injury I gave up sports. But I picked up another one. I played 6 more seasons in the NCAA with my leg the way it was, and boy was that difficult.

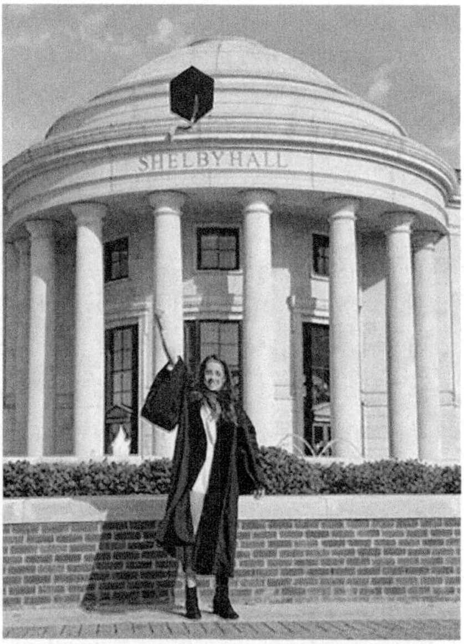

The name's Conte - Doctor Juliana Conte

Towards the end of undergrad, I learned about lymphedema surgeries by doing my own research online and realized I wouldn't have those options in Canada, so I decided to stay in the States. In 2014, I applied and was accepted to the University of Alabama, where I would pursue my master's and Ph.D., conducting original research in their chemistry department and teaching undergraduates. In exchange, I would receive a stipend to cover my bills and health insurance to cover my lymphedema surgeries. I thought if I could just get through graduate school, in a few more years, I would be on top of the world. I thought the surgeries would lead to at least slight improvements in my leg, and I would be a doctor and ready to take on the world. Well, let me tell you, that is not how it went. Yes, I'm technically Dr. Conte, but my body is still recovering from the years of abuse and stress I put it through. I have had 5 surgeries on my leg since my injury. A stent placement opened up my vein but none of the other surgeries have had any obvious positive results. The pain I endured after my omentum transplant in 2019 was something I don't wish on anyone. Not a day has gone by without

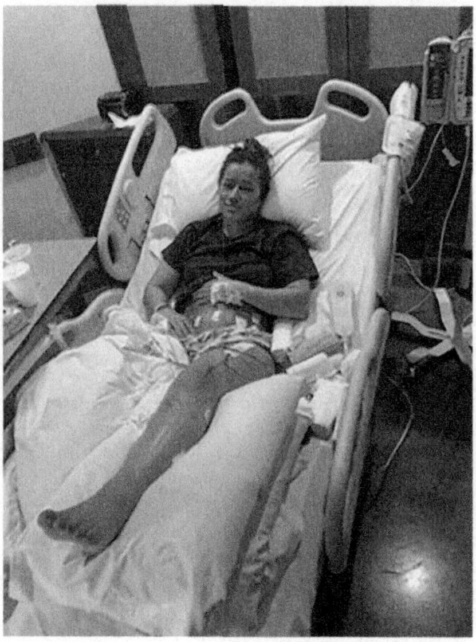

Juliana Conte - Omentum Transplant, 2019

pain in my abdominal area (donor site) as well as increased pain in my leg (implant site).

Over the past 12 years, since I hurt my leg, I have been met with so much resistance. It felt like I was living a nightmare like I was in a life that wasn't my own. And now I realize it's because I was trying to live a life that was not meant for me. All the while, being so resistant to having Lymphedema be part of my identity in any way. In 2016, I made my Instagram account @lymphie.fit and it took a lot of courage to just do that. I posted a picture of my lower legs and started to connect with Lymphies around the world. Some of the first people I met are doing so well in their lives and seem so genuinely happy and that is amazing to see. And some of them don't post about Lymphedema anymore because they're focused on enjoying their lives now that their condition doesn't hold them back anymore. I wish I could be like that sometimes and just feel so free from the captivity of lymphedema, but I'm just not there yet. I'm still in substantial pain daily and sometimes it makes me so angry that I end up making myself feel even worse, and it's just a negative spiral. But I don't ever want to separate my life from the lymphie community, because I have the opportunity to help someone somewhere in the world, every single day. There are people who are suffering from the mental, emotional, and physical effects of Lymphedema, and I want to help them get through things that I didn't think I was going to get through.

There are certain things that I would suggest to other people suffering from lymphedema. Everyone will process and work through things on their own timeline, and sometimes it's hard for us to face a tough reality. I encourage you to face things head-on and stop running away. Running might feel like relief but I promise it won't last. Some people run by pushing themselves harder, and others run by neglecting their bodies and allowing the swelling to progress. The sooner you can stop running and turn around to face the challenge of managing your condition daily, the sooner you will start building a firm foundation for your future. When you are diagnosed with lymphedema you might try to hold onto your past or might be fearful to look into the future. I encourage you to be brave and bold and trust that this condition is manageable. I have seen many stories of people who went years without a proper diagnosis, let alone treatment. When I got my diagnosis, I stayed on top of management from day 1, but my condition has been very severe. Not a day has gone by without multiple different methods of compression, manual massages, deep oscillation therapy, and elevation. If

I slack on my treatments for too many hours, my leg visibly begins to fill up with blood and swell. It's very painful, especially after my last surgery. Things are really tough sometimes, but I have always found a way to survive.

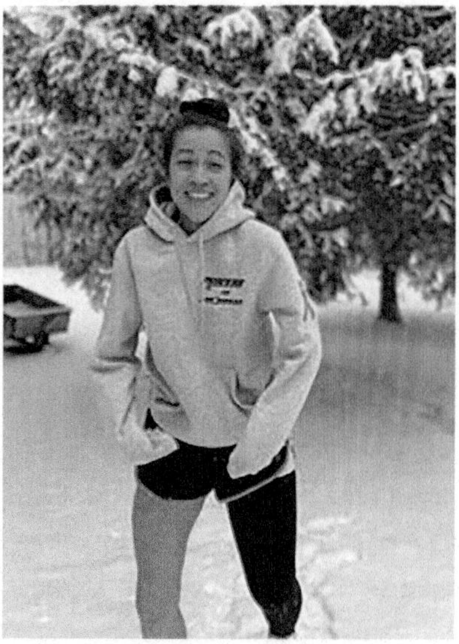

Juliana Conte - I am a warrior!

Physically, I adapted to my new Lymphedema life through the discipline I established many years prior. But mentally and emotionally, I am still working on that. I have always been disciplined. That is what allowed me to manage my condition so well for the past 12 years. But I would be lying if I said that Lymphedema didn't flip my entire life upside down. Lymphedema took me through some of the hardest times of my life. The frustration and devastation come in waves. There were points when I felt myself almost wishing I had the courage to end my life prematurely. But I also always felt a very deep and strong unwavering presence that never allowed me to physically go through with any evil plan my pain was pushing me towards. Lymphedema has tested my patience, resilience, endurance, and finally, my will to live. But now I face it head-on, and I encourage you to do the same. Lymphedema brought a lot of ugly truths about the world to the surface for me. Truths are ever present, but I may not have been exposed to or understood if it weren't for a chronic, progressive, debilitating disease. I see the world for what it is. My empathy, compassion, and love for others is ever growing. Lymphedema proved to me that I can do very hard things, even when simultaneous battles need to be fought daily regardless of how I feel. It has forced me into the darkest corners and forced my faith to grow stronger than it has ever been. The road to where I'm at now has been treacherous, to say the least. And all the while I hid the pain behind my smile, as if my struggle was something to be ashamed of. I realized after the lonely uphill battle, hitting dead end after dead end, I decided, screw this. If I have to suffer this reality regardless, I am not wasting any more energy hiding it. I am relieving myself of the duty to protect other people from my reality. If people stare at my compression or make rude comments, it only tells me that they would never be able to survive my reality. They are too scared to even meet someone suffering, with love and acceptance. I am honored that God chose me to carry this burden and has allowed me to be tested and refined by my struggle. I haven't had a pain-free day in 12 years. Some days I thought my main goal was to escape this misery, but I see more clearly now. I am a warrior, and I will never give up on myself or allow anyone around me to give up. I will continue to pour love and encouragement into this community.

I am so grateful for my leg. My leg has brought so many amazing people and experiences into my life. Remember, whatever you focus on will grow. Don't focus on what you think you lost, or you'll miss all the things you can gain. My leg has taught me so much. I thought I was a loving person before but now my heart bursts at the seams. And there are so many people who are going to feel it. I spent too many years in the darkness, questioning everything about myself. I was lost, but I am so blessed to have been found. If you have lymphedema, you have a unique opportunity at your fingertips. You have the chance to redefine what it means to live with lymphedema. To live well with lymphedema, you need to up your self-care game. That means healthy physical movement, food, sleep, mental rest, compression, and always seeking better ways to take care of yourself.

The other option you have is to run or try to ignore it. I can promise you that it will catch up to you, and quickly. So, save yourself the time and effort of digging yourself out of a hole and start now.

TOP TIP!

To live well with lymphedema you need to up your self-care game and always seek better ways to take care of yourself.

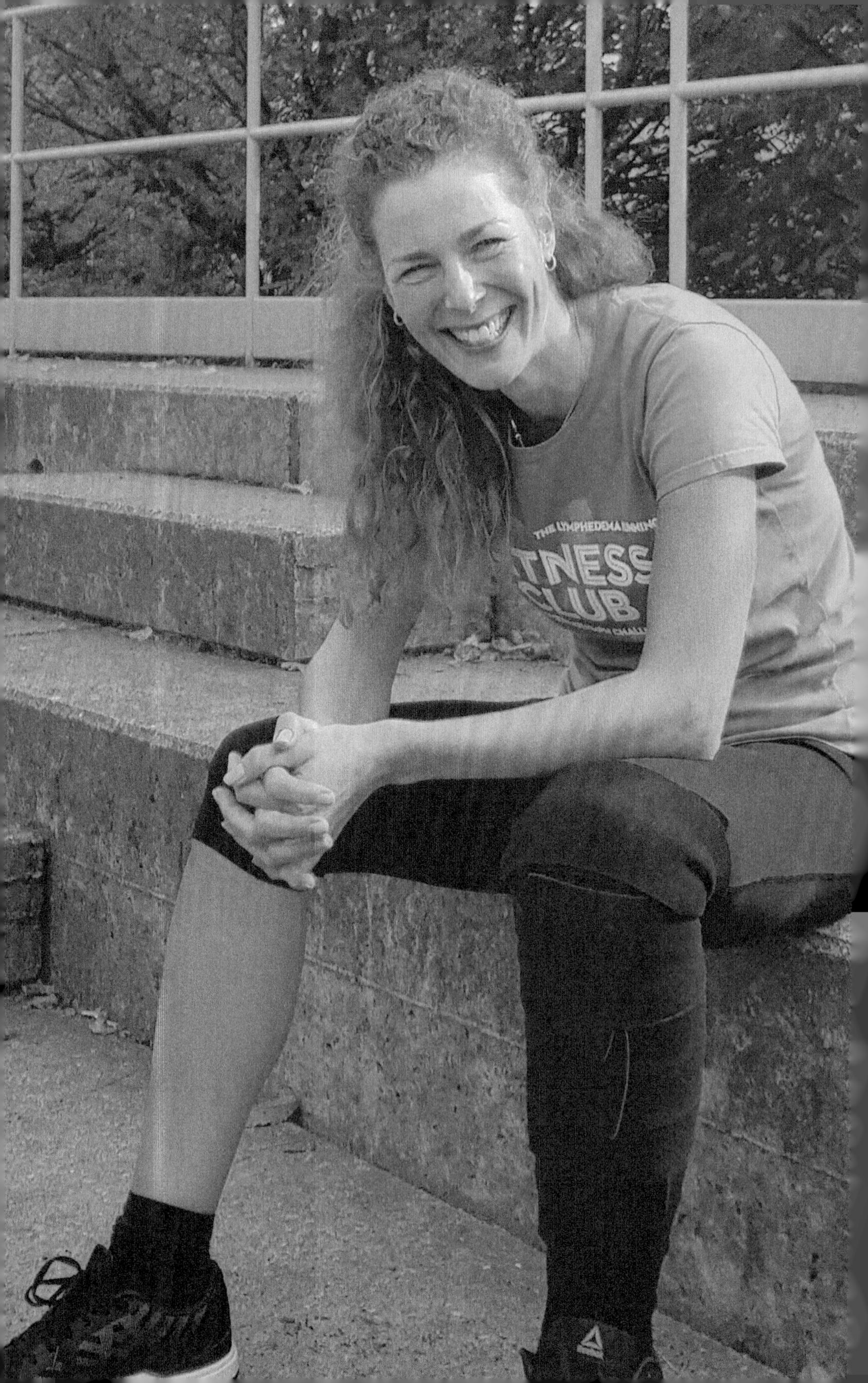
TNESS
CLUB

28

PERNILLE HENRIKSEN

> ***I realised that it was MY leg, and it was MY responsibility. I had to take care of my leg because nobody else would.***

Looking back at my journey with lymphedema I realise that once I started embracing my leg and educating myself, a whole new world opened up for me. A world with a growing caring community of patients and expert clinicians passionate about lymphedema and us.

However, that took many years.

My name is Pernille and when I was about 17 years old, with no clear explanation, my left leg started to swell. Some days it would swell more and other days not at all. Recently I found a picture of the very first time it happened. For those outside the lymphedema world it seems like nothing. Nothing to be alarmed about. And that is why I suspect my GP just told me to do a bit of venous pumping exercise and take some herbal supplements.

This went on for 3 years. Inexplainable intermittent swelling of one foot and lower leg. The swelling got more persistent though, and I consulted another GP who immediately got alarmed and referred me to the local hospital to test for a blood clot. There they diagnosed me with primary lymphedema.

And that was that.

No flyers, no information, no follow up – "just" a prescription for a stocking.

I remember walking home from the hospital thinking that it was fascinating, like a novelty, eager to tell my parents that I had found out "what I had". Like it was a passing disease. I was not the least concerned about skin care, risk of cellulitis, importance of compression, progression.....because I had no idea. I had no idea about lymphedema and what a beast it can be.

At this time, I was studying, working at a record store, partying with my friends and had no interest in this flat knit knee-high stocking I was prescribed. The material was so rough on the skin, so tough in the material and thick. I was not keen on wearing it.

I then started my first full-time job where I worked with a wound care nurse. One day she showed me a book with pictures of legs with severe lymphedema. She pointed at them and said, "this is what will happen if you don't start wearing your stocking". It made a profound impact on me, and I took it to heart. I was prescribed a much "nicer" thigh high stocking which I actually wanted to wear.

And so, I carried on and wore my new stocking.

Until one day, years later, I was on my way to a sales conference with my colleagues. In the airport I started having a sharp pain in my thigh. I thought I had strained a muscle, but I also felt sick, had a headache, felt drained. All day I lay in the hotel room feeling worse as the day progressed. In the evening I finally pulled my stocking off and was alarmed by the redness and the tenderness of the skin. I called some colleagues who got me to the nearest hospital.

I was given antihistamine, as they suspected I had an allergic reaction to my stocking. They kept me in the A&E for hours, until finally the staff was alarmed by my condition.

At this time, they then suspected necrotising fasciitis and I was brought with ambulance for surgery at a different hospital.

Nobody at the hospital had yet made the connection between lymphedema and cellulitis. And I was not able to weigh in on this as I was ignorant. Ignorant about my condition and the risks associated with having lymphedema.

Finally, after more deliberation among 3 surgeons, I was given antibiotics. Lines were drawn on my leg to see if in fact it was responding and if this was the right cause of action.

After my sick leave I went back to work with a new stocking but without prior decongestive (reductive!) therapy. My leg from then on had a new size and shape.

I landed in hospital with cellulitis another two times and from then on, I recognised the symptoms and learned to keep antibiotics at hand.

Besides cellulitis I also had folliculitis quite a few times, pressure sores from badly fitted compression, wounds on the toes as well as leakage from the skin. The compression I was wearing was not suitable nor adequate and my leg, feet and toes were getting bigger, harder, and more difficult to manage.

One winter I was on several rounds of antibiotics. I was sad. I was always hiding my leg under long skirts or large trousers. I could not fit in any shoes. I did not want to talk about it. I always worried about the leg yet somehow never fully embracing it and caring for it.

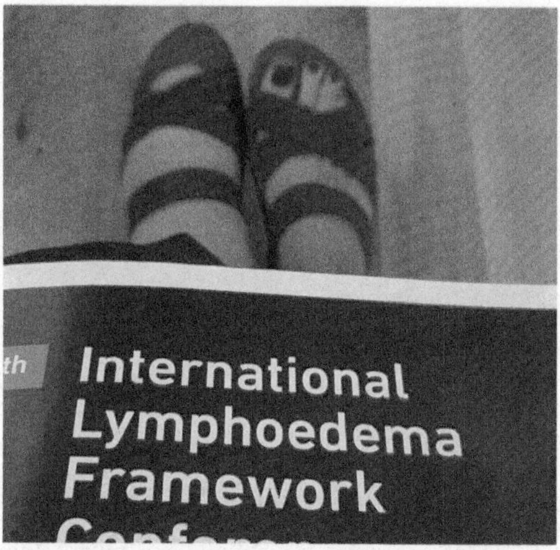

Pernille Henriksen with ILF Conference Brochure

I decided to attend my first International Lymphoedema Framework (ILF) conference in June 2017, and this is where it all changed. As I listened to the experts who passionately talked about patientcare, advances in treatment and manageable solutions, a lightbulb went on.

I realised that it was **my** leg, and it was **my** responsibility. I had to take care of my leg because nobody else would. It took me 23 years to finally accept my condition, embrace my leg and start managing it correctly.

I got my first cycle of decongestive therapy with a lymphedema therapist and a bandaging kit to start self-bandaging. This was the start of my journey.

The 4 key points I have learned along the way to self-manage, as well as educating myself on lymphedema, are:

1 To take good care of my skin including learning the signs and symptoms of cellulitis

2 To move that lymph in any way possible reviewing any flare ups and adjusting accordingly

3 To find support among other patients, and

4 To use adequate and suitable compression.

Compression, compression, compression. I wear it 24 hours a day. I only take it off to shower, swim and to change into another type of compression. I love the feeling of support that it gives my leg. Even in summertime a multilayer bandage will feel like a comforting hug.

I changed from a circular knit stocking to flat knit and got a flat knit toe cap too. My lymphedema is much better managed, the texture of the skin improved, I have less pain and discomfort especially after a long day.

I also started bandaging, a long learning process that I continue to improve. I modify to the mood of my leg and the seasons. I incorporate new materials and learn from those who generously share their tips and tricks, both expert patients and clinicians.

Night-time compression was a real game changer for me. I saw a drastic improvement in my leg, and I sleep much better too. The nights where I have either been too lazy to bandage or tried just wearing a stocking my leg becomes "unruly" and wakes me up. So, there is no good reason for me to skip this vital part of my routine.

Previously I had shied away from exercising because often when I did exercise, I had flare ups. But I realised that it was because I was not wearing suitable and adequate compression. Once I understood this was the problem, I have been able to explore many different types of physical activities.

I have enrolled in several Lymphie Strong fitness challenges with other lymphedema patients from across the world, where we keep each other accountable and benefit from the encouragement of a community of likeminded.

My preferred activity has become swimming, which was something that I used to hate. One reason why I hated swimming was because I had to expose my leg. I feared everybody would look at it, wonder what was wrong. I also worried about donning and doffing the compression stocking in a hot and humid environment.

But now I have devised a meticulous system for both going to the pool and the seaside and I even have a Saturday morning swimming buddy with secondary lymphedema. My system involves among other things good skin care, choosing a pool with not too hot water, a cool down period to allow the heart rate to come down and a well-fitted swimming costume.

I think it is important to find a type of exercise that is suitable for one's lymphedema but also for one as a person. Exercise is not only beneficial for our lymphatic health but also our overall and mental health. Swimming helps me with all of these.

Previously I had not realised or acknowledged how important skin care is. I never took care of my skin but now I moisturise twice a day – with an aloe vera gel before donning my daytime garment and a thicker cream for my night-time bandaging routine. But it is not only the lotions and potions that help me keep my skin in a good shape but also my attention to any cracks, thickening of the skin or even ingrown hair. All things that can lead to complications for me and further aggravate my lymphedema.

Connecting with other patients – both in real life but also virtually – to exchange ideas and support has been fundamental. Not only have I been able to find numerous new ways to manage my lymphedema, but it has done wonders for my mental health as well. We lift each other up on the bad days and cheer each other on for every centimetre reduced or new stocking unboxed.

And the more we connect, the more we can raise awareness and build a stronger patient community.

This journey led me to become not only my own advocate but also advocate for other patients across Europe. I have had the privilege of collaborating with other passionate patient advocates and expert clinicians from across Europe. Including some of those who presented at the ILF/ITALF conference in Siracusa in 2017 which kick-started my journey.

You can follow me on Instagram @the_lympha or join me on the Lymphie Strong groups online.

TOP TIP!

Join a national patient association. The patient associations work hard to improve the conditions for those with lymphedema and raise awareness with medical societies, the policy makers and the public - so please support them. You can also find likeminded patients in Facebook groups or on Instagram to exchange ideas on how to live better with lymphedema. You are not alone.

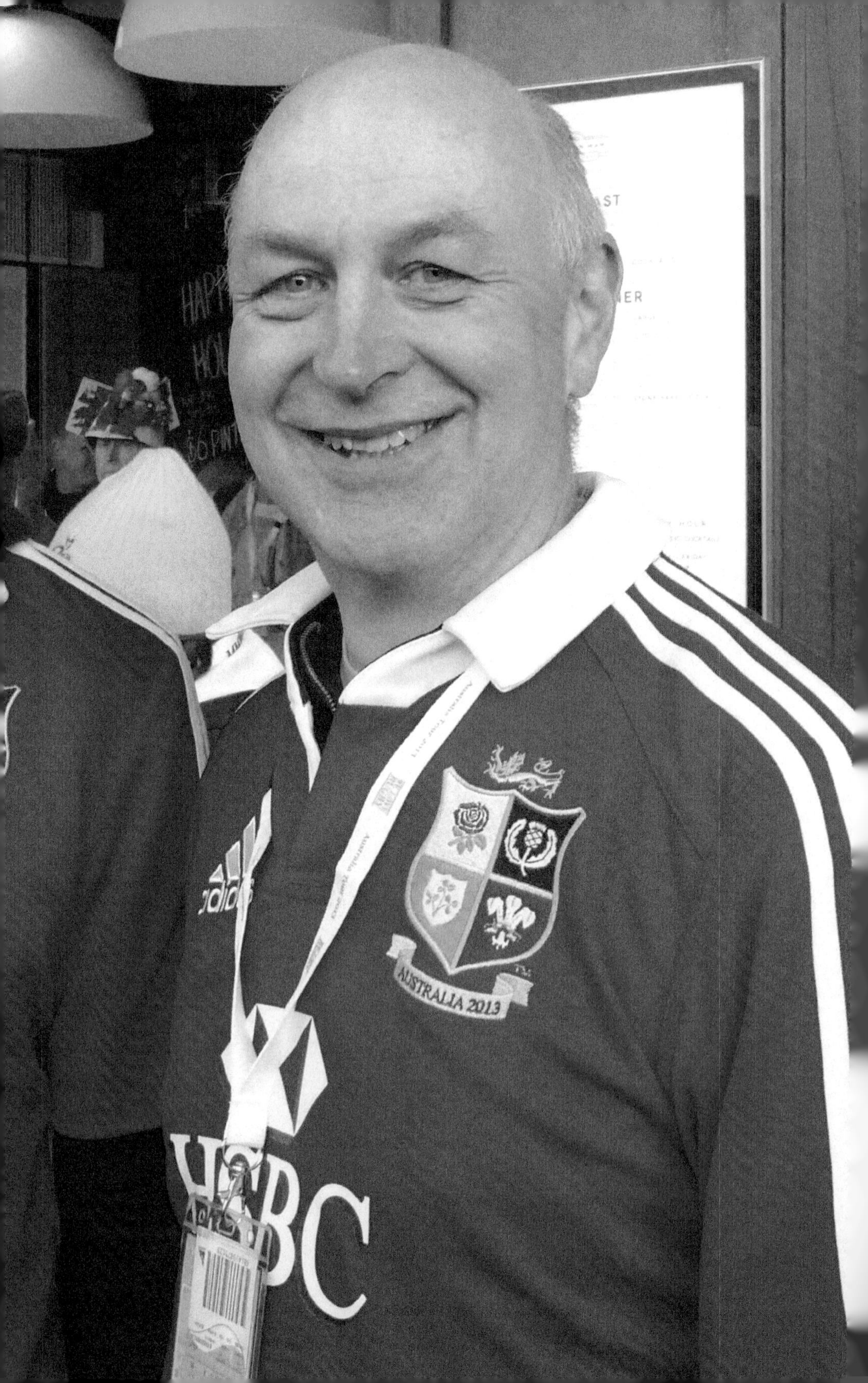
AUSTRALIA 2013

29

ROB WILLIAMS

> ***I have not bottled these things up. The specialist nurses at Prostate Cancer UK were, are, absolutely brilliant, and helped me out of a number of dark places.***

Lymphoedema entered my life on 17 June 2019, although at the time I had never heard of the word, let alone the condition, nor did I have the slightest inkling I had it or what was to come.

At the start of the winter 2018-19, I decided to see my GP. For the third winter in a row, I found myself running to the loo all too frequently and enough was enough. At the time I worked for a hospital charity and my line manager was the fundraiser for prostate cancer, so I had read all the leaflets and I did not have any of the major symptoms. I had never been offered a Prostate-Specific Antigen (PSA) test, even though I was 57. Two PSA tests later, one a bit too high, the other even higher and I was off to the hospital for an MRI scan. 'We've found an anomaly in your prostate and have taken the liberty of booking you in for a biopsy' said the letter. The day after my biopsy, I was rushed by ambulance, with blue lights flashing to Accident & Emergency (A&E) and spent the next six days in hospital with sepsis and a positive diagnosis for cancer. On 17th June I was on the operating table having the offending bit removed, along with a couple of otherwise now redundant bits, and 36 lymph nodes.

This was not how retirement was meant to be. Thirty years as a police officer ended with compulsory retirement, but with only two days' sick leave in the last fourteen years. At this point I took a bit of a detour. Autumn 2019 saw me doing my first little jobs in the garden after my operation. The most awful stomach-ache hit me and I had to lie down for a few hours. The same happened the next day. A few days later, on a short break to Norfolk with my wife, an ex-nurse saw me get another attack. I almost passed out. "You've got gallstones" announced my wife (the ex-nurse) who was somehow enduring these episodes with me. True, she was right. February 2020 saw me back in hospital having another faulty bit removed.

Six months after the cancer operation, I was pondering why my groin felt squidgy. I had more important things to worry about, the two things that every man facing a prostatectomy obsesses about, incontinence and impotence. The only two things, strangely enough, that are constantly drawn to your attention before the operation. There was no third, no lymphoedema. The leaflets said the wound could take six months to heal, 'I'll mention it at my nine-month review if it's still the same', I thought. The nine-month review, March 2020, never happened, because Covid did!

Therefore, due to lockdown restrictions, all my reviews took place on the telephone. During one call with my GP (Doctor), I told him about my groin, "Just lymphatic fluid draining" he announced airily, in a matter-of-fact manner that effectively dismissed my fears. Even so, I really felt the urge to cross my legs whilst sitting down. I know you should not, but when you cannot, you really want to.

In April 2020, I started work as a bank porter/courier at a local hospital. Yes, that's right, one month after Covid arrived I went in to cover for the staff who could not work. I thoroughly enjoyed it until late November 2020. I went into work feeling under the weather, I could not put my finger on why, but I did not feel 100%. I felt as though I'd strained something in my right thigh. During the night I woke up and instantly thought, "I have the flu". I ached in every joint. The next morning all of those aches had gone except one, in my right shoulder. I also had a raging temperature. Somehow, I drove to the Covid testing station then went home to bed. I was not the most popular person in the world. My little grandson had decided to make his entry into the world and my wife was due to babysit our granddaughter, instead she was isolated at home with me. The next morning, I felt worse but at least it was not Covid. Throughout that day I got worse and worse. The pain in my shoulder was excruciating and I could hardly move it. Strangely, my groin and right thigh had gone red. After hours of waiting on the phone to the 111 NHS helpline, I was granted a phone call with a doctor. He asked if we could do a video call. Within thirty seconds of seeing my shoulder and groin I was on my way to A&E.

Twelve days in hospital followed. The doctors were baffled. The fluid aspirated from my shoulder revealed nothing and they just waited for the inflammation markers in my blood to reduce. Septic arthritis, nobody was in the least interested in my groin. Eventually they operated and removed a part of my shoulder, another bit I did not need. Discharged, I was back at A&E a couple of days after completing the antibiotics. I was put on double strength antibiotics for a week; two days later I was back at A&E. Both times I just generally felt yuck, under the weather and had a high temperature and a red groin. And that, in a nutshell, describes 2021. I felt just like that every fortnight for the whole of the year. To be fair to the GP he fought a battle with the hospital, explaining 'you cannot just discharge someone like this.' The NHS spent thousands of pounds on fancy tests. Whenever we discussed symptoms I told them, I feel yuck, have a high temperature and my groin and thigh go red. At this point the doctor would put his/her chin in his/her hands and say, 'how weird.' The doctor from Infectious Diseases had her eyes light up, "Have you been abroad?", "Yes". "Do you always go with your wife?", "No". "Aha, where have you been without her?", "Africa". "And did you have unprotected sex whilst there?", "No!". Except she did not ask once, but many times, which was uncomfortable and frustrating to say the least.

By the late summer of 2021 I was getting fed up. Going to work was problematic, family days out were problematic. Would I feel well enough? Would I have a temperature? (Remember, having a temperature in 2021, during Covid, was very problematic, especially every fortnight. I felt like a leper. I had to lie). At this time, and all of a sudden, my groin felt much worse. It felt much more full, much more squidgy. I sat down with my wife and we had a full and frank conversation. "Remind me exactly what they did when they took out your prostate" was the killer question and the moment the lightbulb came on. It was also the day that,

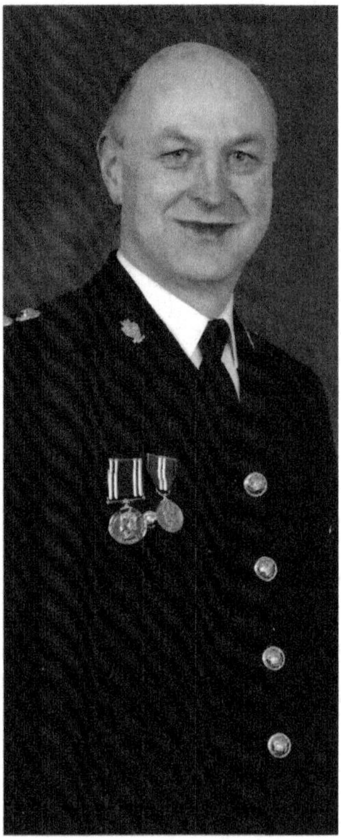

Rob Williams -
Thirty years as a Police Officer

suddenly, things got a lot better. It has its benefits being married to an ex-nurse!

They obviously took out the prostate with both 22mm tumours, they removed the vas deferens, the seminal vesicles and 36 lymph nodes. "The technical term for a collection of fluid after removal of lymph nodes is lymphoedema" she said. It pains me to say it but on such matters she is usually right, remember the gallstones? I went straight onto the NHS website. Things are so much better when you know what to Google, believe you me 'swelling in the groin' does not reveal the same results as 'what is lymphoedema?.' Eureka! I had the key and it was turning the lock.

When I was waiting for my cancer diagnosis a good friend, Tina, who had just been diagnosed told me that waiting was worse than knowing, even when it was positive. I totally agree. Now I had a name and I could read about what was wrong, equally I had places to go. I could tell them that I had lymphoedema and cellulitis. I told the doctors and they agreed.

I have not bottled these things up. The specialist nurses at Prostate Cancer UK were, are, absolutely brilliant, and helped me out of a number of dark places. I rang the Lymphoedema Support Network and they sent me details of a nearby specialist. All of my recent illnesses have taught me one thing, do not rely on the NHS alone. My specialist is called Karen and she runs The Lighter Touch in Malvern. Despite the fact that within a few days of contacting her I was in her treatment room stripped off whilst she showed me how to bandage 'my bits' and how to massage my groin, I can honestly say that everyone needs 'a Karen.' At first Karen and I tried to manage my cellulitis not only through massage and exercise but also through changes to my diet and supplements. Ultimately, that did not work and in February 2022 I went onto daily antibiotics, but the gap between attacks had spread out to three weeks and the changes I made to my diet have stuck. I see Karen every four to seven weeks and apart from the physical help she provides mental support, through talking and listening. Mind you, when she first applied Kinesio tape to my groin I did remark, "I hope I don't get carted off to A&E like this they will think it's some bondage fetish!".

The world of compression garments was also something very new to me, although they are now second nature. It would now feel very strange to get up in the morning and not put them on. The same as not doing my massage after going to bed. Because my lymphoedema is in the groin, raising a limb is not really an option. I find that my ordinary, everyday life complicates my lymphoedema whatever I do. Sitting down for long periods leaves me feeling very heavy in the groin. Equally, so does standing up and walking around. I have come to accept that I feel heavy no matter what I do during the day, that is now part of my life. I try to break up my day between walking, sitting and standing. I also try to fit in other exercises, such as cycling. I have been recommended to take up swimming but that has a big mental barrier of cold, crowded, public swimming baths to overcome! It is not an activity I enjoy. I have also struggled to find suitable exercises for me. Everything I see on the web is aimed at limb exercises. Finding specific exercises for the genital area is defeating me so I am using leg exercises from an online yoga course. In fact, finding anything out about compression shorts is difficult. Even looking at manufacturers' websites you struggle to find them. Doctors especially ask if I'm wearing 'stockings'. I ended up lodging my first complaint about my GP over my compression garments. And my second. And third. And fourth. Events unfolded in exactly the same way each time. I would submit the prescription request, knowing it would take two weeks to make them. Just as the two weeks were up the GP would phone me, "There's a problem with your garments. You have not given us your measurements." I would tell them I had, they would find them, the garments would be made. The GPs did uphold all my complaints and hopefully the problem is rectified.

My cancer treatments and my lymphoedema have been intertwined all along the way. Whilst I am not incontinent, I am however 100% impotent. The tablets do not work, the vacuum pump did but it messed up the lymphoedema, so had to go. I have few options left. It can have its funny side. Attending a clinic to see the urology nurses (they are always female), the guidance stated to wear loose clothing because of the reaction you may have to the medication (how coy).

Loose clothing? What's that? As I undressed in front of the nurse and her student they remarked, 'those shorts look great' and my Mobiderm shorts do look good and it is welcome to have a medical garment that looks nice. I have lost count of the number of females who have now peered intently at my bits, or is it 'for' my bits? Better that than the reaction of my, male, GP when I first asked for Viagra. "Have you discussed this with your partner? She may be relieved." Give me female staff to discuss my problems any time.

Despite all of this I do not regret having had the surgery. Ultimately, I am still here. I did not have a choice, radiotherapy was not an option, but even if it had been, it too risks causing lymphoedema. At present it is not stopping me living my life. I had to give up one job because I was on my feet all day, virtually standing still for ten hours and this was when I was having my cellulitis attacks. I felt very heavy and weary by the end of the shift and after a cellulitis attack my scrotum would swell to the size of a grapefruit. I have had to give up running, so my plans of a half-marathon with my daughter went out of the window. I still do a lot of walking and I enjoy getting out watching nature. I still plan holidays abroad. I think I have another safari in me, and I still plan to go to South America on bird watching trips. I just have to pay more as I am not prepared to do long-haul in economy class anymore. This means I still have to look for work, which is fine by me, as I still enjoy going out and mixing with other people.

I have no real magic wand to offer other people. My main tip is to remain open-minded. Be prepared to talk about your problems and be prepared to try anything. Only by trying things can you find out what works and, just as importantly, what does not. I have managed to get my NHS Trust to use the British Association of Urology Surgeons' (BAUS) notice to men who are due to have a radical prostatectomy. This does at least mention the risk of the 'collection of lymphatic fluid.' Today I have heard that the BAUS plans to include the word 'lymphoedema' in that notice after I made the request to them. Men will now be forearmed with some knowledge.

TOP TIP!

Remain open-minded. Be prepared to talk about your problems and be prepared to try anything.

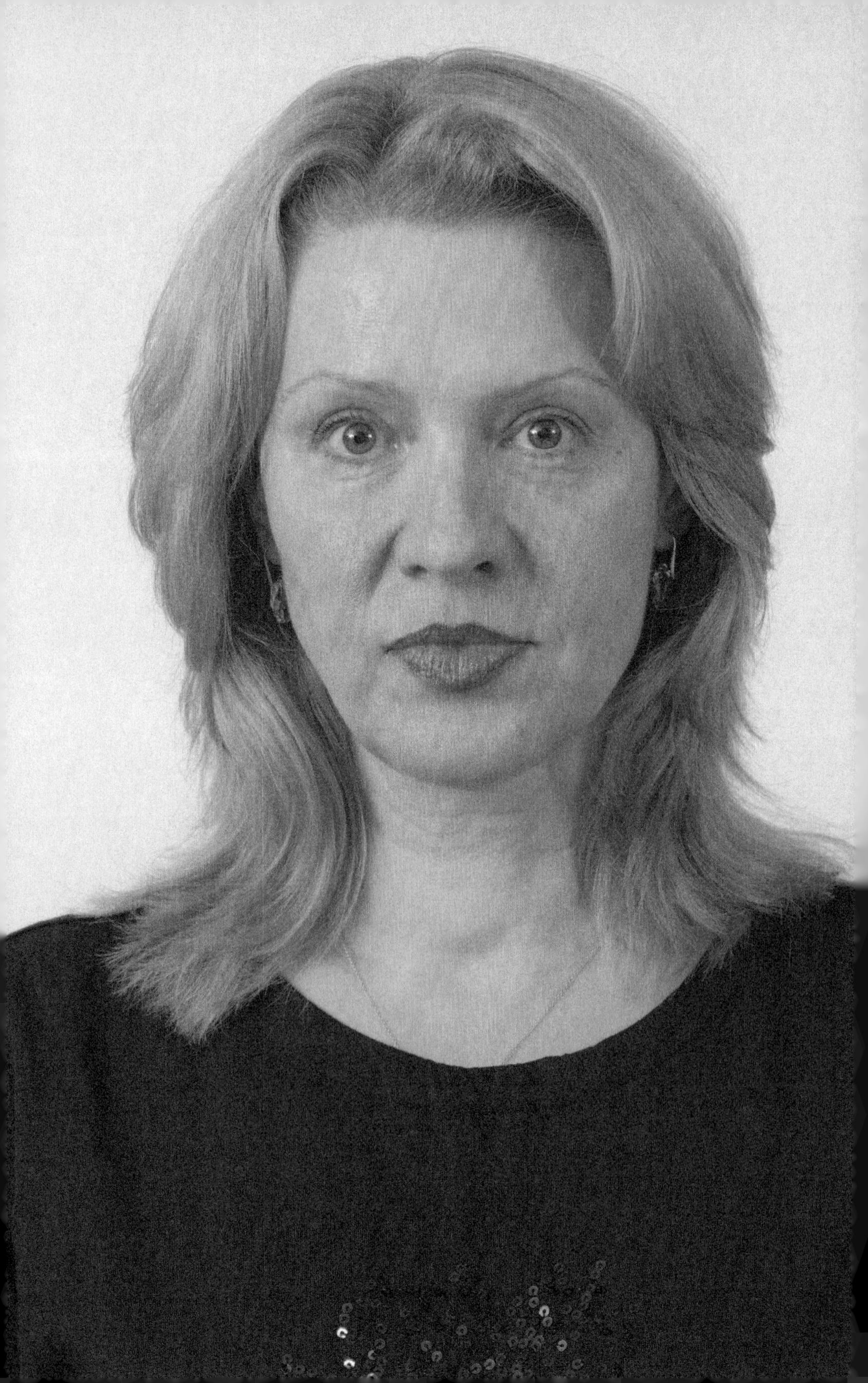

30

PETYA STOYCHEVA

> ***Gradually I found that controlling the physical impact of the lymphedema was very effective in reducing its emotional burden.***

I am a patient with secondary lymphedema on my right leg, after cancer surgery in 2011. My lymphedema appeared almost immediately as swelling on my inner thigh. I did not know what lymphedema was and I was not informed of its possible occurrence as a side effect of treatment. The very next day after its appearance I was in my oncologist's office looking for advice. Even though he had been dealing with similar situations for years, he had no idea how to help me. He prescribed me pills to improve venous flow and told me it was a "cosmetic defect" that I had to learn to live with.

In the beginning, the lymphedema kept appearing and disappearing, fooling me into thinking I had dealt with it, but with each new appearance, it went further and further down my leg. Back then there wasn't so much information about this disease, even on the internet, whereas today there is plenty of adequate advice. I had no idea it was progressive and would get worse with time. Most of what I found about lymphedema was limited to pictures of people with huge, misshapen limbs that were so startling, but I had no idea how they had gotten to this state.

I went from doctor to doctor, but all I heard was there was nothing to be done, no treatment. I was told to accept it and learn to live with it. I couldn't agree with that. I couldn't believe that in the 21st century, where everything is evolving at such an incredible speed, there is no information anywhere on how to deal with a swollen foot. I started looking for information in all languages on the internet. It was, of course, still very sparse but I still found out that I needed manual lymphatic drainage, a low-salt diet, exercise, and compression clothing.

I had to look for solutions and find out what helped me on a trial-and-error basis.

Manual lymphatic drainage was offered everywhere in beauty salons, but I quickly realized that it was not what I needed and that I needed a qualified medical professional. The problem was that there were no such specialists in our country. Even today (May 2023) there is still not a single specialized lymphedema treatment center in Bulgaria.

Physical activity worsened my lymphedema because I was not wearing the right compression garment. I did not know this at the time and for this reason I chose to rest instead of exercise for a long time, which in turn further worsened my condition. I felt like I was in a vicious circle, but I understood that the way to get out of it was to educate myself. So, I kept searching for information and putting it together piece by piece. It was like I was making a puzzle.

I went through pills to improve venous flow, skin creams, and gels, pressure therapy machines (I even bought one, a budget version of the professional machines). I also joined a yoga class and swam during the summer season. I wore a compression sock, but with a circular knit because there was no other option available here. Since my lymphedema started at the top of my thigh and went down to the bottom, standard drugstore socks didn't do the job. If I purchased a size that was comfortable on my thigh, it was necessarily wide on my ankle and caused swelling. If I picked up a size that would hold my ankle tight, it would dig into my thigh and the area above the sock would become hard. It was also painful and uncomfortable to wear.

Although I sometimes achieved relatively good results in the care of my foot, they were very unstable. The moment I stopped my daily efforts, the swelling would return even greater than before.

So, in late 2016, a little over 4 years after surgery, one day my foot swelled all the way from top to bottom and never came back. None of what I already knew as information was helping to get it back to its previous state.

The search for a way to stop the progress of the disease led me to a small group of Bulgarian lymphedema patients on Facebook who, like me, were trying to solve their problems. In the summer of 2019, some of us created an Association of Lymphedema Patients in Bulgaria. Our aim was to try to draw public attention to this much-underestimated problem and to seek help and support from institutions.

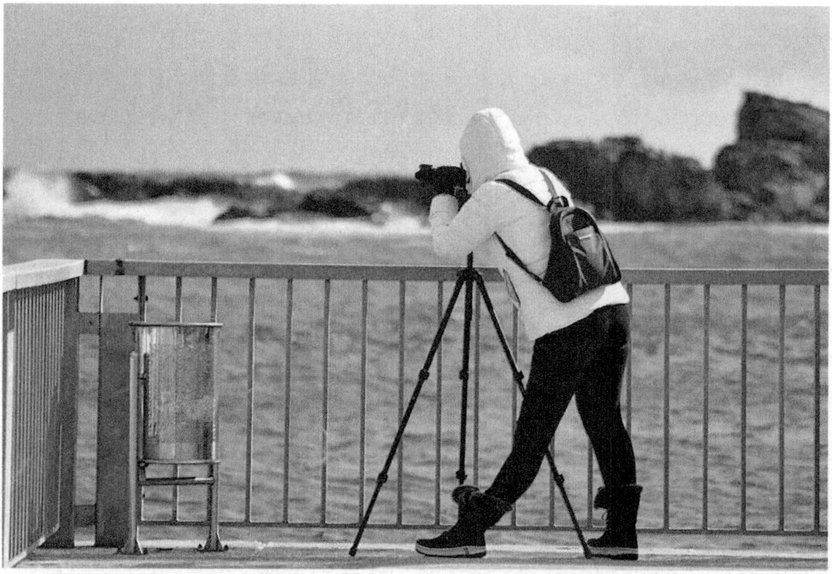

Petya Stoycheva controlling her condition and returning to a normal life.

One year later, the covid-19 pandemic completely changed the face of awareness on the internet. The restrictions on live meetings made it necessary to hold many international events online. So, in September 2020, I came across an international conference on lymphedema organised by Dr Alexandra Rovnaya. The two days that I was glued to the computer screen gave me those missing pieces of the puzzle that I had not been able to find on my own over the years. I now had the answers to questions like – 'Why doesn't manual lymphatic drainage work for me?' 'Why doesn't a compression sock stop my swelling?', 'What is a compression garment made of flat knit?', 'Why do my leg swells when I exercise?', etc.

Since we already had a connection with the importers of one of the leading compression garment brands in Bulgaria, we requested them to start importing flat knit garments as well. For the standard in Bulgaria, the prices of compression garments are extremely high and unaffordable for the majority of patients, yet the fact that we can now order them from here was a huge step forward.

In March of the following year, our association, together with Dr Aleksandra Rovnaya, organized and ran the first online training meetings for lymphoedema patients. Later that year, I met Aleksandra in person in Romania, where I attended the Decongestive Therapy Specialist Training course, she was running there for five days.

Ten years after the beginning of my lymphedema, I was finally in a place where I was surrounded by people who understood my disease and knew how to help me. We often talked about solutions instead of resigning myself to the fact there was nothing I could do. I felt a sense of security and peace that I hadn't felt in years. I will always be grateful to Dr. Rovnaya for that feeling and for the humanity he showed toward me.

I still continue to learn every day. There is now an ocean of information to dive into and find what works best for you. I started by ordering two low stretch bandages (how naive of me to think they would be enough to make a bandage) from a site in Australia. I now have a huge collection of bandages, various pads for under the bandage, foam, low elastic systems, night compression garments, pamper pads, knee pads, and a bunch of other stuff from various companies that I use to manage my lymphedema. And of course, compression socks with flat knit. I wear them all the time. They're made to my size, manage to keep the swelling in my ankle down, don't dig into my thigh and don't cause pain.

I don't always manage my lymphedema effectively, although there isn't a single day I don't wear compression. There are days, especially in the summer season, when it is very hot and my work is too busy. Then I just don't have time to take good care of it or I'm too tired. There are days when I don't feel like long walks or active physical activity. Of course, on such days my foot swells more than usual, but I don't panic anymore because I know what to do and I go back to my routine at the first opportunity to reduce the swelling. I have learned to do my own lymphatic drainage, which is effective. I have learned to do self-bandaging with low stretch bandages when higher compression is needed. It was very difficult at first, but as time went on, this care became automated and took less and less effort.

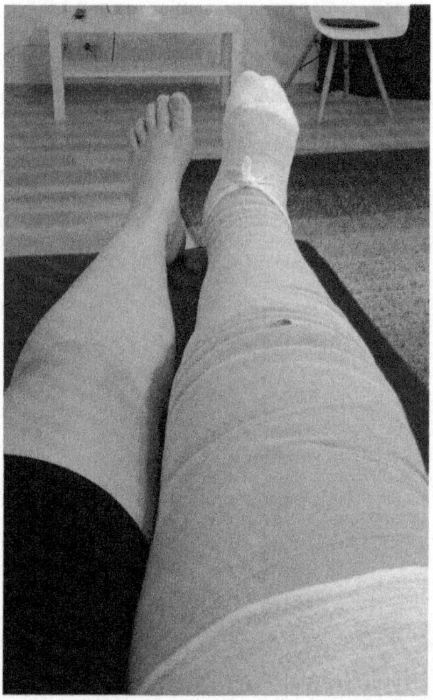

Petya Stoycheva in Multi-Layer Lymphedema Bandaging

I realized that it was much more important to maintain the functionality of my affected leg and to protect myself from bacterial infection or other complications, than to try to make my legs uniform in shape again. Although I haven't entirely given up on that goal either.

I also continue to actively volunteer with our patient organization. Having successfully removed the information curtain regarding lymphedema in Bulgaria, our next goal is to get the support of the state. We need trained specialists, lymphedema treatment centers and reimbursement for compression garments. To this end, we are also partnering with other European, lymphedema-related patient organisations with whom we exchange experiences, ideas and support each other.

More recently, we have also become a member of the International Lymphoedema Framework, and in this way we hope to be able to contribute to international progress in the development of care for this disease. Because we believe that quality information should be shared and because we believe that together we can achieve faster and better results in finding a solution.

During the years of trying to deal with my problem, I have learnt many things that has changed me in a more positive direction. They have taught me to be more patient and gentle with myself, to be less critical and more loving of myself. Perhaps the hardest thing in the beginning for me was dealing with the emotional burden that accompanies illness. I was experiencing a wide range of emotions – fear, anger, rage, frustration, embarrassment and depression. Gradually I found that controlling the physical impact of the lymphedema was very effective in reducing its emotional burden (and the financial burden as well, which is not to be ignored). The more I learned to control my condition over time, the more relaxed and confident I felt to return to my normal life. Focusing my efforts on the things I can do, rather than on what I can no longer do, is probably what still helps me the most in my daily life.

TOP TIP!

Be patient and gentle with yourself. Focus on the things you can do, rather than the things you can't. Both can reduce the emotional burden of lymphedema.

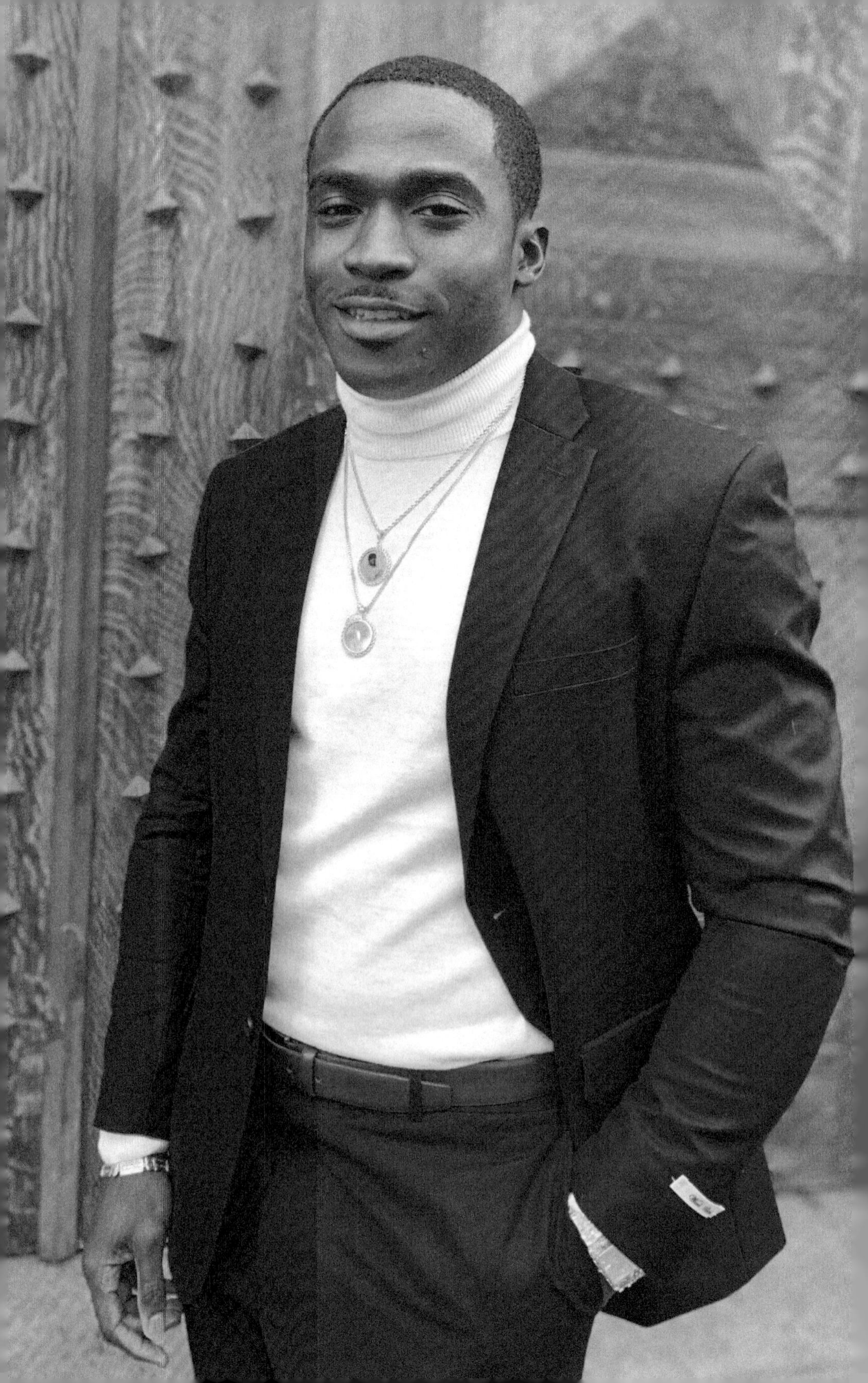

31

DOMINIQUE ROGERS

> ***Lymphedema has created a new purpose for me in my life, and I intend to carry out that purpose, for myself and for others.***

My name is Dominique Rogers. I am 34 years old, and I was born and raised in Hartford, Connecticut. I currently reside in Hartford and work for the city as a firefighter.

When I was asked by Amy to write a chapter to include in this book, I thought hard about what I wanted to write about. Ultimately, I decided to write a little about everything and give you a brief overview of what my life has been like for the last 20 years.

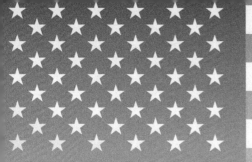

Growing up I was a very active kid. I played outside with my friends and participated in sports enjoyed riding my bike, and even used to race with my friends whenever I could. However, the life that I was used to completely changed when I was 15. On a hot summer day, I was outside playing basketball and rolled my ankle. What seemed like a minor injury quickly turned into something more serious. When I got home, my mom advised me to elevate and ice my swollen ankle, but the next day, my entire leg was swollen. My parents brought me to the hospital, confused and filled with anguish about how something as simple as rolling my ankle could cause so much inflammation to my leg. Laying in the hospital bed at that moment, I thought to myself, I'm sure there is a reasonable medical explanation for what was happening to me, and once they figure it out, they can cure me. What initially began as a one-day stay in the hospital, turned into three, turned into a week; at this point, as an inpatient teenager, I was ready to leave and go home. Eventually, me and my parent's questions were answered when a doctor came into my hospital room and told me, "You have a condition called Lymphedema." He began to explain what it was, and my only question for him was, how do you get rid of it? He told me there was no way to get rid of it, as there were no procedures to remedy my condition, and I would have to wear a compression garment for the rest of my life.

Before being diagnosed with lymphedema, I had never heard of the condition, didn't know what it was, and certainly didn't know anyone diagnosed with it. I felt very alone and angry that this was happening to me. I couldn't believe that of all people, it had to be me, and that there was no cure for this. I would be stuck this way for the rest of my life. I thought about things that I wanted to do, like possibly going to play college football, and I felt that dream getting further and further away from me. My first year living with lymphedema was one of the hardest years of my life. When I was in the hospital, the doctors explained the consequences of not taking diligent care of my leg.

They also explained that I could become more susceptible to certain infections in my leg due to this condition. During that first year, I caught my first case of cellulitis. It was one of the most painful things I had ever experienced up to that point. Beginning with soreness in my leg, my leg would also get red and hot. I felt a shooting pain that would run down my leg. I would get a high fever and chills. This would result in hospital stays that would last days, sometimes even weeks. I could hardly walk, let alone stand for long periods of time. I realized then that my condition would not be going anywhere, and this was something I would have to endure for the rest of my life.

After a few years of living with lymphedema in my life, I now had a better understanding of what my condition was and how I could manage it. I knew what to do, and what not to do, to keep my leg healthy and free of any infections. I began to see a lymphedema therapist down the street from my home, whose goal for me was to decrease the size of my leg. Therapy has and continues to work very well for me, along with the support from my family.

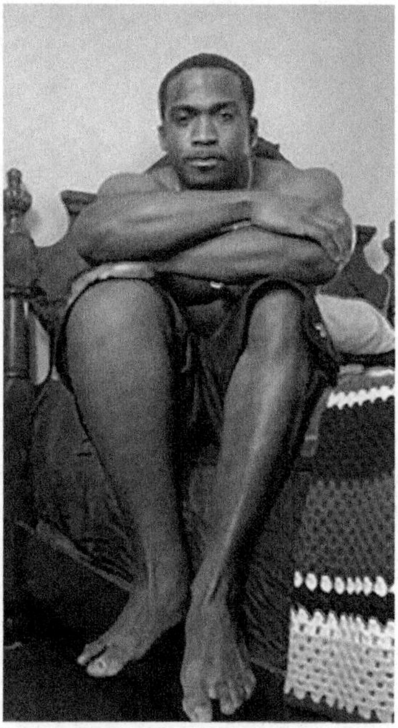

Dominique Rogers - I know what to do!

My biggest supporter, and the person who was there with me through it all was my mother. I was a mama's boy growing up. I hugged my mother any chance I got, kissed my mother on the cheek any chance I got, and would bring her flowers any chance I got. My mother was the cornerstone of our family. She is the strongest person I've known. She was a God-fearing woman who walked by faith. I was always close to my mother, but little did I know that life would bring us even closer. One day, when I came home from school, my mother and father called on me and my brother and told us that they had something important to talk to us about. She calmly explained to us that on her doctor's visit that day, she was notified that she had a cancerous mass in her breast. I immediately began to worry, and I could feel the tears begin to swell in my eyes. At that moment, I remembered something my mother always told me, something that has stuck with me throughout the years. She said, "When the doctor says one thing, God can say another."

As she began treatment for cancer, her doctors advised her they would be performing a procedure in which they would take her lymph nodes out of her left arm to stop the spread of cancer in her body. In turn, this could potentially cause her to become diagnosed with lymphedema. I thought to myself, there is no way this could happen to her. But sure enough, one day after I came home from school, she called me into her room. She sat on her bed, with lymphedema in her left arm, looked at me calmly, and said, "I'm just like you now." I immediately began to cry, and we embraced each other. I felt as her son that I wanted to be her protector and seeing her go to cancer and now Lymphedema I felt that there was nothing I could do. However, my mother being the strong, faithful woman that she was, continued to fight, and that motivated me to continue to alongside her. I was already a mama's boy, but this only deepened our bond. We were a team.

We had each other's back, supported each other, and helped one another to manage our lymphedema the best that we could. I would help put her compression garment on as she got ready for her day in the mornings. She made sure that I would go on my compression pump machine at the end of my days before I headed to bed. We also went to therapy together. My faith was a big component of my coping because she instilled that in me at a young age. One of her favorite scriptures is Hebrews 11:1; "Now faith is the substance of things hoped for, the evidence of things not seen." My mother always told me to not give up on anything I do, especially as someone with Lymphedema. Unfortunately, my mother passed in 2015 from her battle with cancer. She fought a good fight and I miss her every day. Her legacy lives on through my love for her and all that she has taught me throughout the years.

In 2020, I decided that I needed to tell my story about my life with lymphedema, because I realized that I could help someone else going through what I had gone through. One day I made a post on Instagram talking about lymphedema, including what I had overcome and accomplished in living with my condition. In my years of living with lymphedema, I became a full-time firefighter, a part-time EMT, and a business owner. I knew that there could be someone else who would benefit from hearing my story, and I could possibly inspire them to continue pursuing any dreams or goals that they had for themselves. To my surprise, in the last 3 years, I have gained an immense amount of support and positive feedback from my very first post from people all over the world. It was soon thereafter that I realized there was an entire community of people with lymphedema on social media. I've been lucky to meet people from all areas and walks of life, fighting the same fight I'm fighting.

One day while lying in bed I realized, there was a process I had to go through to get from the day that I was diagnosed, to the place I, after everything I had been through, came to the place I was at in that moment. That's how I came up with the awareness brand, Process To Progress. My purpose for this brand was to help people who couldn't afford compression garments for their lymphedema, while simultaneously promoting awareness for lymphedema, and letting other lymphedema patients, like me, know that whatever you want out of life you can have, if you are willing to go out and get it. Everything takes time, everything is a process! My goal for Process To Progress is to continue to raise awareness for lymphedema and raise and donate money to help people obtain compression garments that can't afford them, and motivate and inspire people who have a dream they want to accomplish.

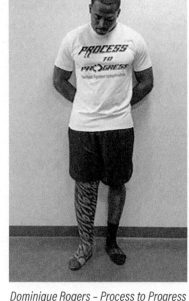

Dominique Rogers - Process to Progress

In the next 5 years, I want to host a walk for lymphedema in my state and invite others with lymphedema, as well as supporters, to walk for the cause. I would also like to create a scholarship fund for students who inspire to go to school to become lymphedema therapists. I believe that through my brand I can make a huge impact in the lymphedema community.

Looking back at my journey with lymphedema, there are many things in my life that I never thought I'd be able to do. At 15, I would have never thought I would be talking to people about my condition and how I've been able to accomplish my dreams. I would have never thought I would be an advocate. I would have never thought I'd be the recipient of LEARN's 2022 Courage Award, one of my greatest honors. Finally, I never thought that I would be able to connect with so many people all over the world. My ability to accomplish all of this, and more, has come from my consistently positive mindset. Through all my hardships, I never once gave up on myself, even when I wanted to. Lymphedema has created a new purpose for me in my life, and I intend to carry out that purpose, for myself and for others.

As I was writing this chapter, I wanted to close it out by including some advice for anyone who has just recently been diagnosed. First, be patient with yourself. The first year will not be easy, but you will get through it. Second, on days when you feel like giving up when you question why this is happening to you, have faith. Have faith that things will get better because they will. Have faith that you will continue to pursue your goals and dreams because you can, and you will. Seek out a lymphedema community online, or lymphedema support groups near you. It can be scary to meet new people at first, but you will begin to feel less alone in your fight and more motivated to continue to keep fighting. Remember that the good days will outweigh the bad. Continue to take care of your health and remain health conscious. Lymphedema becomes incredibly easier to manage when you are taking care of yourself physically and keeping up with your doctor's and therapy appointments.

TOP TIP!

My mantra, everything takes time, and everything is a process!

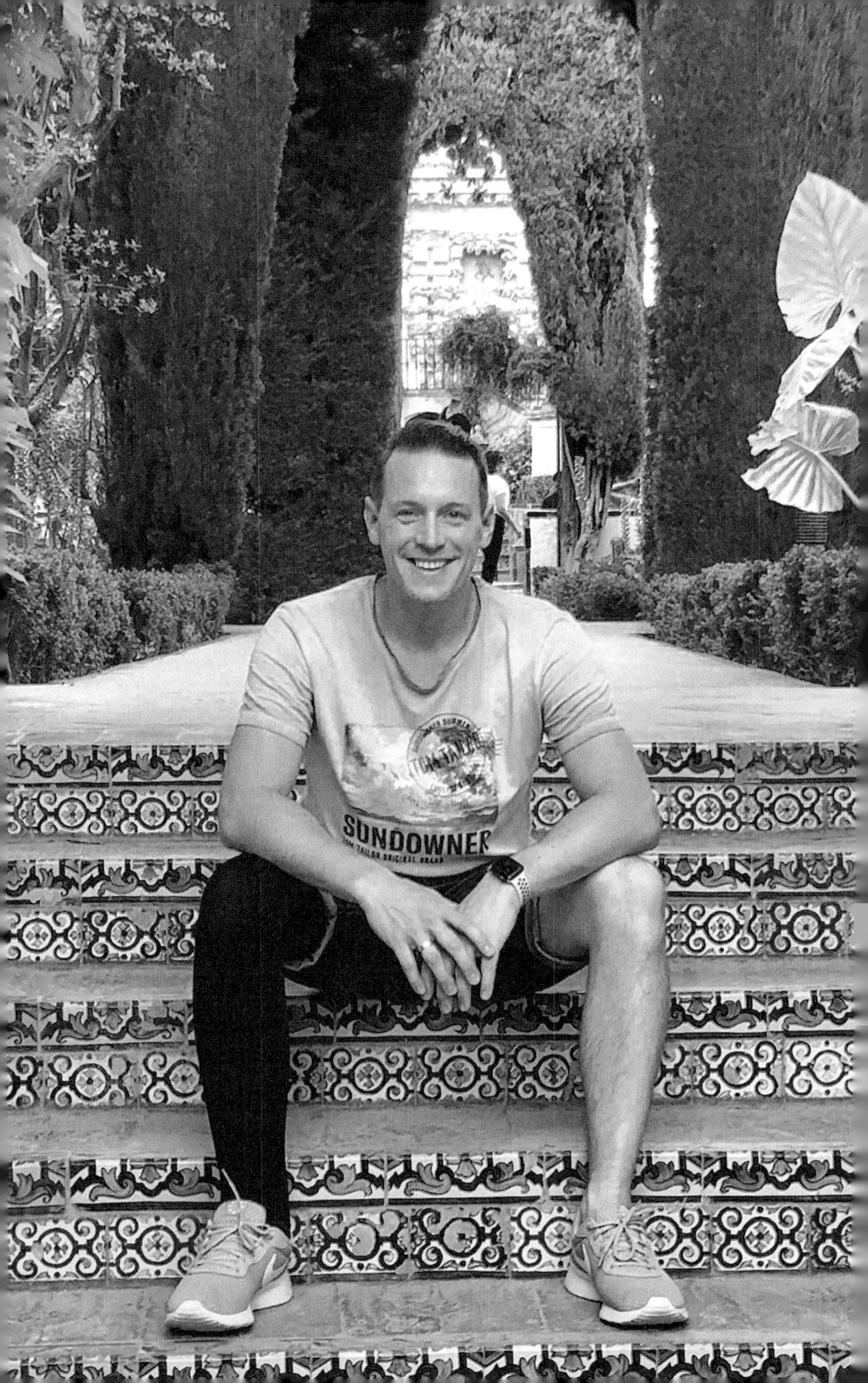
SUNDOWNER

32

PIERRE HASPEL

With the right support, dedication, and self-care, you too can manage your lymphedema and live life to the fullest.

Reflecting on my life, I realize that my history of lymphedema has been intertwined with my personal growth. From a young age, my parents noticed that one of my legs was consistently thicker and more bulging than the other. It wasn't long before I was diagnosed with "primary lymphedema" at a renowned university clinic in Heidelberg, Germany, shortly after my third birthday.

The recommended therapy at the time involved regular lymphatic drainage sessions and the permanent use of medical compression stockings. The diligent application of these treatments yielded positive results, providing me with much-needed support in all aspects of my life. It was during the summer of 1989, just before my sixth birthday, that I embarked on my first rehabilitation experience at the Földi Clinic. This marked the beginning of a journey where my lymphedema

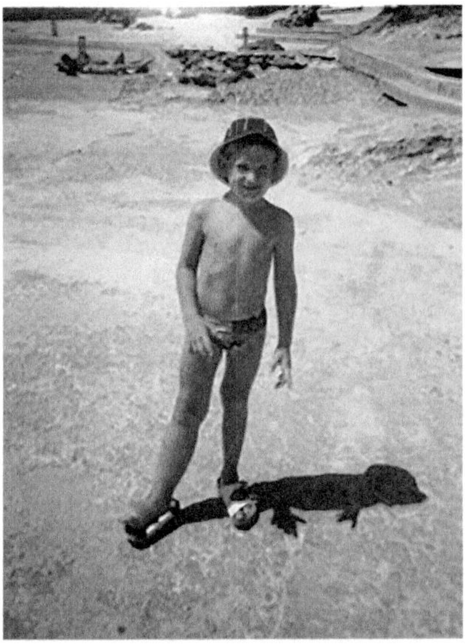

Pierre Haspel - It was the Summer of '89

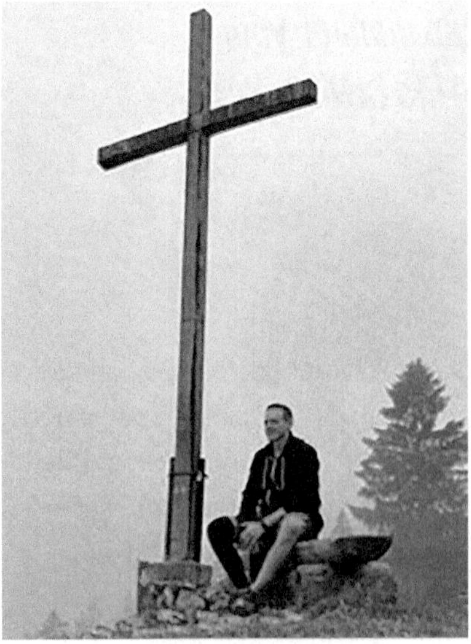

Pierre Haspel - Keep the faith

was well-managed, and I experienced relatively minimal challenges for years to come.

However, as I approached my 18th birthday, a brief setback occurred when my leg condition worsened due to erysipelas, a superficial skin infection. Determined to regain control, I sought rehabilitation once again, this time at the Földi Klink Hinterzarten. With their expert care, I successfully managed the infection and resumed pursuing my greatest passion: sports. Throughout it all, I remained committed to my compression therapy, which played a vital role in my daily routine. Today, I rely on class 3 compression stockings, along with a body part and toe cap, to effectively manage my lymphedema. I must say, the results have been very positive, and while wearing them daily requires discipline, it is absolutely manageable. The best part is that I have been able to maintain my condition without the need for any medication. Looking at it pragmatically, one could say that things could have been worse.

Nonetheless, I continue to prioritize my well-being by undergoing regular rehabilitation sessions every 3-4 years. These visits ensure that my edema remains stable and prevent any further deterioration. I cannot stress enough the importance of finding a skilled therapist and wearing perfectly fitting compression garments for every lymph patient. In addition, adopting a healthy diet and incorporating regular exercise into your routine can work wonders in keeping your lymphedema under control. These seemingly time-consuming measures are simple yet highly effective.

Wishing all fellow lymphies the best on their personal journeys.

TOP TIP!

Remember, with the right support, dedication, and self-care, you too can manage your lymphedema and live life to the fullest.

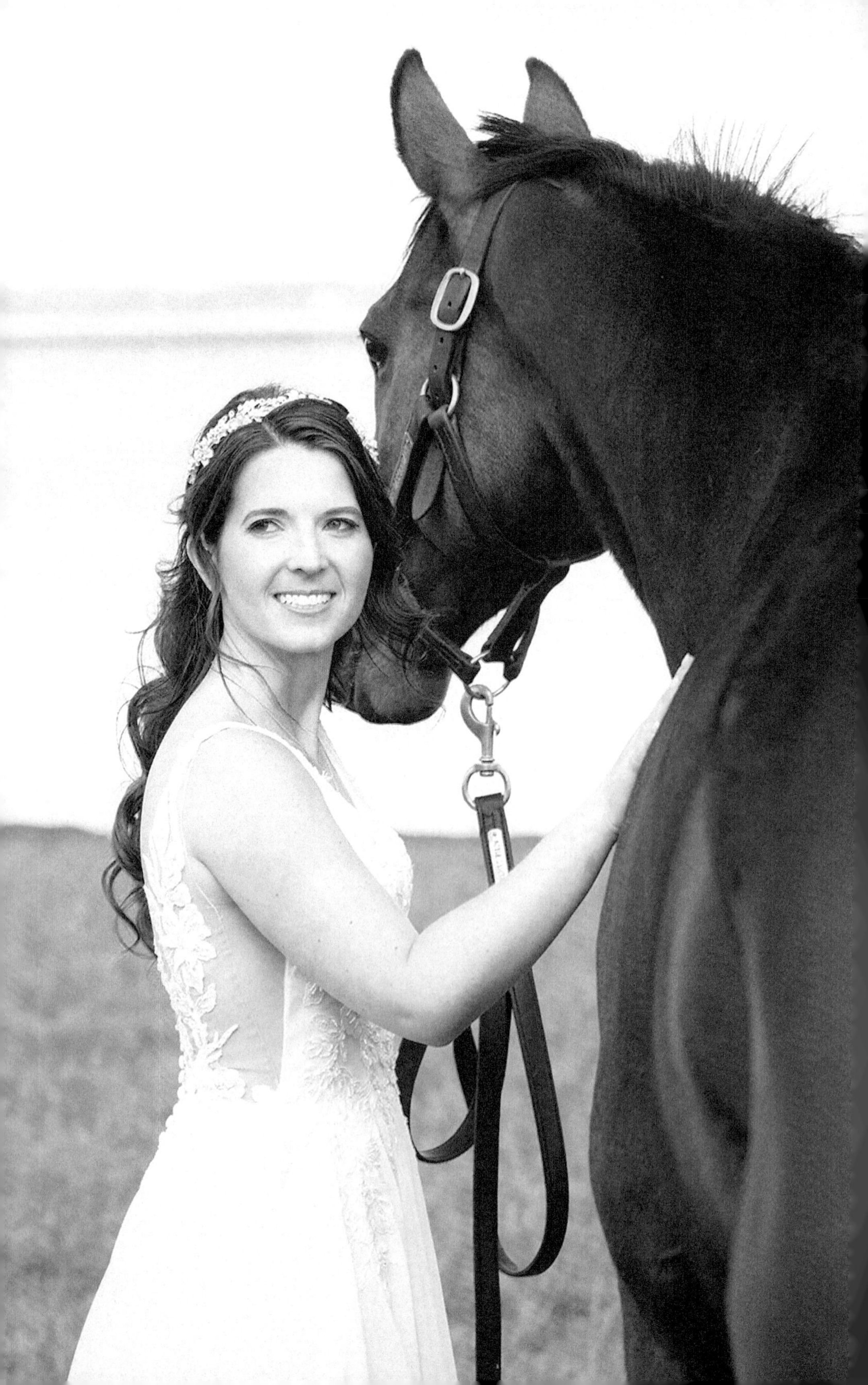

33

KIERSTEN WALL

> ***I became miserable being miserable. I realized something needed to change, and I didn't want to be that person anymore.***

Imagine being your average teenager – in college, weaving social scenes, finding your niche, and discovering who you are. Now, throw in an unknown, incurable disease that affects every second of your life. That's me. My name is Kiersten Michelle, and I am thriving with Bilateral Primary Lymphedema. This is my story.

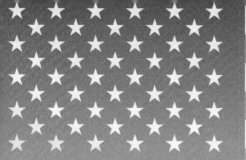

My story began with unresolved localized swelling in my right ankle at the age of sixteen. Unfortunately, nothing was found, so nothing was done. With the knowledge I have now, I have no doubt in my mind this was the early signs of Stage 1 Lymphedema. Life went on. At the age of nineteen, a period of sixteen hours changed my life forever. I was a stressed college student, playing NCAA softball, and had no idea what I wanted to do in life. One morning, I woke up with a profusely swollen right leg. It was red, tough, and pitting, and I was incapable of putting pants on. Talk about a curveball. Sixteen hours is all it took to turn my life upside down.

As a college student, I didn't have the time to handle doctor visits to find out what was wrong with my leg. It wasn't broken and our athletic trainers were stumped. I decided to finish out the semester before figuring it out. Meanwhile, daily activities became more difficult. My leg got heavier. The skin was constantly splotchy, red, tough, and filled. After softball activities, there would be muffin tops of fluid hanging over my knee. It was gross and embarrassing, not to mention concerning. Why is it that my body is doing this to me? The summer came along and so did the shuffling of doctor visits. After nearly two dozen appointments, ultrasounds, x-rays, genetic testing, and a fine needle aspiration biopsy I was finally diagnosed with Lymphedema. The specialist's words were, "You will have this for the rest of your life. Here is your referral to an Occupational Therapist." Naturally, I was in denial and searched for other opinions. The crazy thing is every doctor said, "I don't know what Lymphedema is, so I can't help you. I am sorry."

To this day I still see the same therapist, and she is a saint. My first impression of her was that she was the nicest person ever. My mom went with me to the early appointments. She learned how to wrap my leg in bandages and boy was this a comical scene at home. Thinking back, it was hard to grasp the concept of the enormity of the disease; the science of compression, garments, bandages, night garments, skin care, exercise, and manual lymphatic drainage. There was so much to learn about the day-to-day operations of taking care of myself. I remember my therapist saying that the garment will eventually feel like a second skin. After nine years I don't know if I'd quite say that, but I will say my legs feel significantly better with compression than without.

The next four years were full of grief and denial. My leg was huge, my dreams were crushed, and I was down more than I could ever be. I didn't take care of myself as I should have. Not because of excuses, but because I simply didn't understand. I didn't understand the disease and I didn't understand the necessity, nor could I manage my time. It was a challenge to pass my classes and get through each day. Because of sleep apnea, I also wasn't sleeping. What got me through this extremely difficult time was not myself but a small group of peers and my supportive family. I was absolutely miserable and so uncomfortable in my own skin.

I don't know how to explain it, but it's hard work being miserable. I became miserable being miserable. I realized something needed to change, and I didn't want to be that person anymore. For four years I put myself in a deep, dark hole with no intentions of ever coming out. I was angry, upset, confused, and discouraged. I finally said, "Enough is enough" to the bad attitude and my unhappy lifestyle. I had the support, but at the end of the day, it was me that had to take care of my body. Mentally and emotionally, I was stuck in a deep, dark well rinsing with water. There were hands reaching down (family, friends, even strangers) trying to help. However, those hands couldn't reach me without me equally wanting to get out of the well. I had two choices: I could either allow the Lymphedema to slowly drown me over time, or I could reach up and find a way to grab the hands of those wanting to pull me out. After several years of drowning, I finally chose to reach up for the heavens and get pulled out of the well. I became my own saving grace and my life has been so much better ever since. I purchased books, created a Lymphedema Instagram, and I educated myself on this disease. I finally took care of my body. After graduating college, I moved back home and became more focused on taking care of myself. I base my life around taking care of my Lymphedema, not the other way around. I have the commitment and diligence to properly care for my body. My advice is to respect the disease and make the sacrifices needed for your health. If it means not going out or getting the laundry done, then so be it. Despite having help along the way from my husband, it truly is a full-time job taking care of myself – mentally, emotionally, and physically. Utilizing all my tools for my decongestive therapy it's a minute-by-minute routine. There are twenty-four hours in a day. Of those twenty-four, I spend sixteen hours physically caring for my legs or thinking about how to prepare for the next part of the day.

Knowledge is power and no one can take that away from you. This knowledge opened doors and opportunities to begin my surgical journey. I first learned of these operations through other Lymphies on Instagram. My acceptance of the disease also led to more conversations in my personal life. My parents would talk about me a lot when others would ask, "What's wrong with Kiersten?" My father had conversations with in-laws, one thing led to another, and he found the surgeon that would change my life forever; Dr. Oluseyi Aliu, another Saint who came into my life.

Finally, here was a board-certified doctor who could answer five years' worth of questions, confusion and give clarity. At this point, I had been dealing with my Lymphedema for five years and was finally getting proper testing for the lymphatics. A Lymphoscintigraphy and ICG lymphography became my ticket for scheduling my first surgery. I'll be honest, I could probably write a whole book on my surgical journey: the good, the bad, and the ugly. The good is that I have had tremendous improvement. I have a better quality of life, and my legs are healthier. The bad part is the financial burden and difficult insurance processes. The ugly, being totally transparent here, is constipation after surgery.

At this point, Lymphedema had set into my left leg, turning my diagnosis into Bilateral Primary Lymphedema in 2017. Thankfully, by this time, I had the knowledge and knew the signs. Despite going through denial all over again, I had the tools to start taking care of this new edema. In 2019 I had the lymphovenous bypass surgery on my right leg. In 2020, I had liposuction in my right leg, and one liter of fluid was removed in addition to the lymphovenous bypass surgery in my left leg. My legs were doing so well, and I had perfected my routine and mindset to take care of the swelling. In 2022, Dr. Aliu said he was moving hospitals from Maryland to Pennsylvania. That would mean twice as far of a drive for me, but I couldn't imagine putting my life in anyone else's hands. There was no question. I was moving hospitals to continue being his patient.

Lymphedema is such a strange and mysterious disease. As someone with a bilateral case, I would certainly say it is different in each leg. My right leg, my bad leg for many years, has always had the most issues with my calf being the "problem area." On the contrary, my foot and ankle are the "problem area" for my left leg, which was manageable until the summer of 2022 when it changed drastically and became my bad leg. At that time, the lymphography test showed the lymphatics were completely shot and unworkable. This determined my next stop to the operating room for the lymph node transfer from the omentum to the left lower extremity and lower extremity liposuction.

Wednesday, December 14, 2022, I woke up from the sixteen hours that would change my life forever. Eight years ago, my life changed in a negative impact. This time, Dr. Aliu, spent sixteen hours with me on the operating table hard at work changing my life for the greater good. I woke up in the ICU confused, in a significant amount of pain in every square inch of my body, and absolutely starving. I asked my nurse when I could have dinner. (I thought it would be Tuesday evening because the surgery was planned to take eight hours). I will never forget his reaction, "Dinner? It's 3:14 in the morning." My response was, "Morning? What DAY is it?" That's when I learned my surgery took sixteen hours. My mom and fiancé were the only ones in the waiting area all night long.

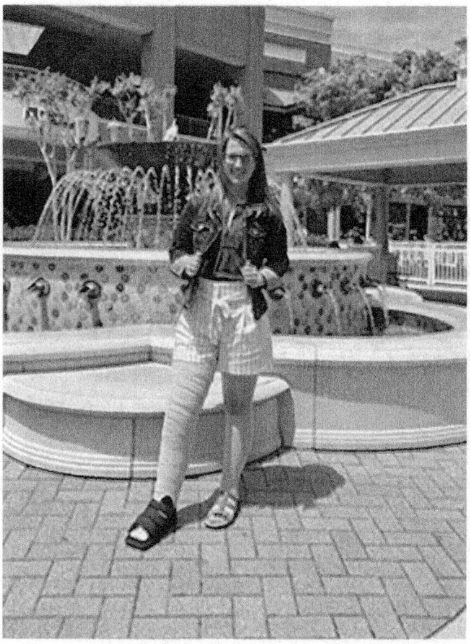

Kiersten Estes - You wear it well!

My surgery took so long because part of it didn't go as planned. So, instead of leaving it as is Dr. Aliu redid the connection putting it in a different location. He was much happier with the outcome of this, so the extra eight hours were well rewarded. This made his job harder, but he wanted to make sure I was one hundred percent taken care of and given the best possible outcome I could have. To say I am thrilled with my results thus far is an understatement. The pain was a long recovery, but it was well worth every minute of it despite how agonizing it was at times.

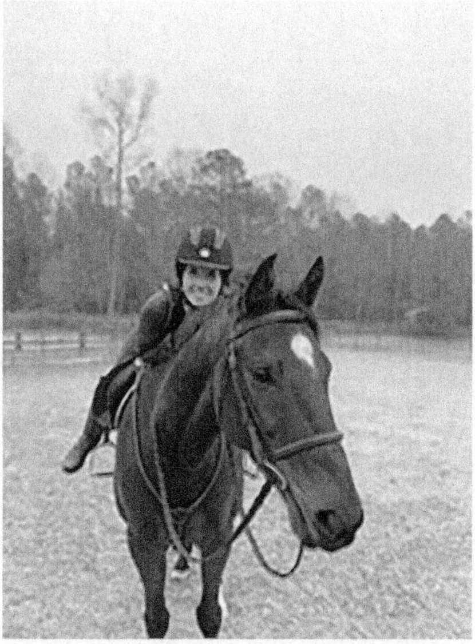

Kiersten Estes - Making tomorrow better.

Because I had to travel several states away, I stayed in an Airbnb with my mom and fiancé through my first post-op appointment. This was by far the best and smartest thing we could have done! I packed everything I needed to stay as comfortable as possible. Not just at the Airbnb, but in the car ride as well. In addition, the most important thing packed was my "leg bag," an airplane carry-on suitcase. This has been the most helpful trick for all my travels. It can hold all my compression garments, one set of bandages for both legs, gloves, tape, and lotion. The handiest part is the pockets that I can use for extra supplies. Forgetting anything when traveling is detrimental because Lymphies can't just go to the local convenience store to get what they need for our Lymphedema. This has saved me so many times.

Every day my goal is to do what I can today to make it a better tomorrow. My life drastically changed when I decided for my mindset to change. That was something that was up to me and me alone. When I made that decision, everything got so much better: mentally, emotionally, physically, and socially. I truly believe the tide can change as long as you're willing to go against the waves. For so long, I fought against the waves of anger, denial, and depression only to get knocked down. Once I became more willing to accept what is I have been able to enjoy the calmness of the open sea. Thus, so many times, in a matter of sixteen hours, my life changed for the greater good.

TOP TIP!

Acceptance is Key

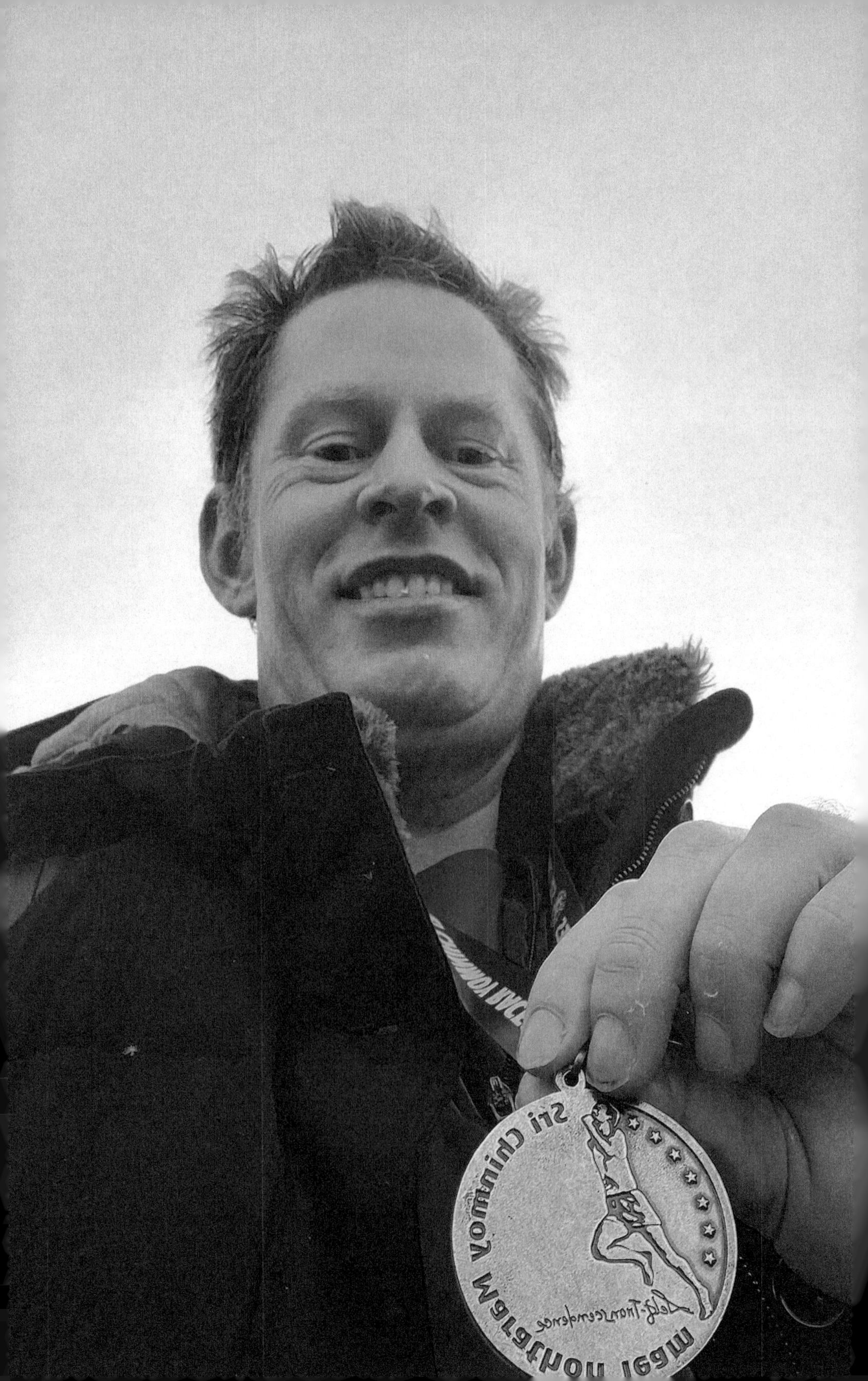
Sri Chinmoy

34

LEONARD VAN BROEKHOVEN

> ***I sometimes find it hard that I have to wear these stockings for the rest of my life. I also am bit ashamed of it and always wear long trousers.***

My story with lymphoedema starts when I was 20 years old. I was on survival weekend when I was at college. After I came back, my left foot started to get bigger. After a week, the swelling didn't reduce, so I went to see my GP. The strange thing was besides my foot getting bigger, I didn't have any other symptoms (like fever). The GP thought the cause was an infection from streptococci bacteria and I was prescribed antibiotics.

I was referred to hospital for further research and I was then diagnosed with secondary lymphoedema. The hospital provided me with compression stockings and for the next 20 years the situation stayed quite stable, besides an infection in summer 2006, where I had to stay 5 days in hospital receiving intravenous antibiotics.

Unluckily, my condition worsened 5 years ago. My left leg got bigger and bigger. In 2019, I went to all different kinds of medical specialists, but there wasn't a solution.

I needed some antibiotica cures, because my leg got infected much easier than usual. That was, until the moment came I met a very experienced and specialized physiotherapist in oncology and lymphoedema. She had a connection with the specialistic lymphoedema center in the north of Holland, called hospital Nij Smellinghe in Drachten. After more research they came to the conclusion that I have primary lymphoedema and not secondary lymphoedema, as first diagnosed.

They did lymphoscintigraphy scans to see the quality of the lymphatic systems in both my legs. It was visible that my right leg was also not good. They also recorded several measurements of the perimeter of my legs, in order to calculate the volume. By the end of 2019 I had 7 liters more volume in my left leg than my right leg.

At the end of 2019, I had an operation called Circumferential Suction-assisted Lipectomy (CSAL) and stayed 4 weeks in this specialist center. The result of this operation was a reduction of 4 liters out of my leg.

At the moment I have 2 liters more and I go back every year for check up to this hospital.

My doctor is Robert Damstra. He is leading doctor in Holland for lymphoedema. After the operation I got stockings for whole leg class 4and class 2 extra for lower leg.

I sometimes find it hard that I have to wear these stockings for the rest of my life. I also am bit ashamed of it and always wear long trousers. The compression the stockings give me is bit uncomfortable.

I got back to fitness and started gently for the first couple of weeks with some walking and biking. I have been doing intensive fitness for 25 years and this has helped me both physically and mentally.

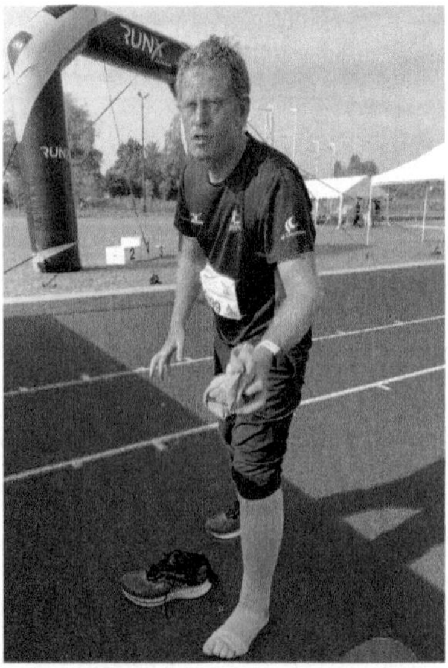

Leonard van Broekhoven –
"I felt better physically and mentally."

I started intensive running 10 years ago, with a friend twice a week. Before this time, I didn't like running at all and I found it even more of a problem because of the stockings and the lymphoedema.

However, after some weeks of doing running, I began to like it more and more. I can say it was life changing. I felt better physically and mentally. I experienced that it also had a positive effect on my lymphoedema. Running stimulates the muscles and lymphatic vessels.

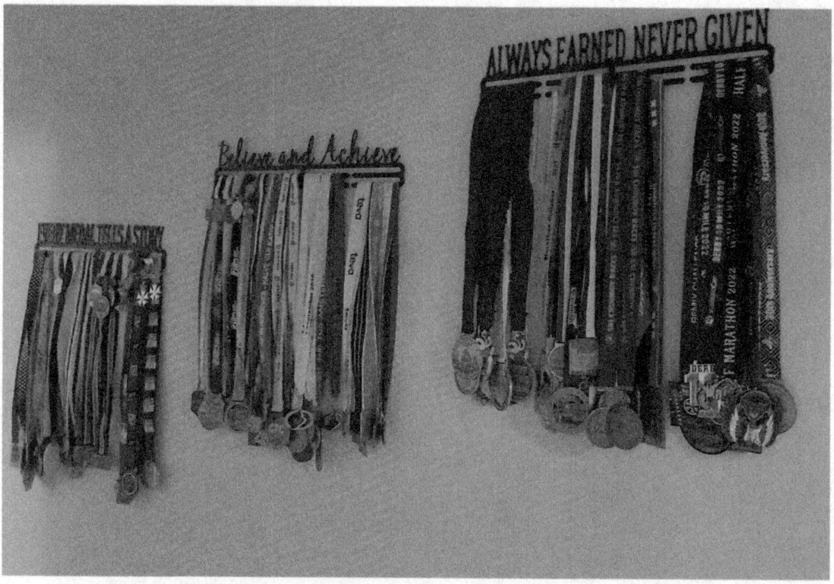

Leonard van Broekhoven - The Marathon Man!

In September 2013 I did my first half marathon and many half and full marathons would follow. Another good thing about running is that it also outside. I hope to motivate other people to exercise more and for them to see lymphoedema as less of an impairment.

TOP TIP!

Try to have optimistic mind set and don't let yourself be impaired by anything or anyone.

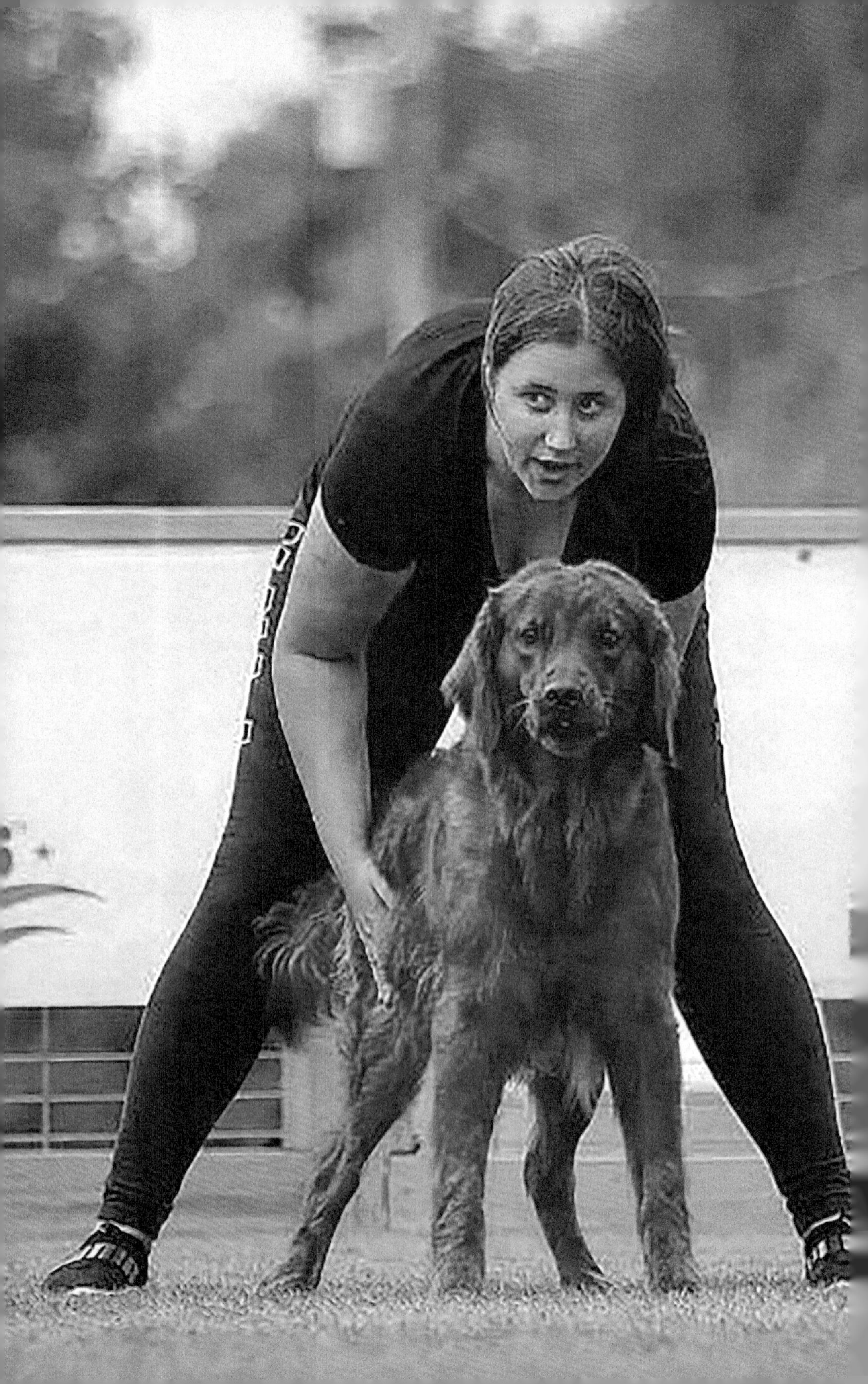

35

JADE GRONBORG

> ***My mother (Amy Rivera) has taught me a valuable lesson—to embrace my journey, to love my body, and, most importantly, to love myself.***

My name is Jade Gronborg, and I was diagnosed with stage 2 lipedema when I was just 15 years old. It was a moment that changed my life forever. While I never felt alone in my struggle, there were times when I felt a deep sense of shame and insecurity about how I looked. Little did I know that within my journey, I would find peace, fulfilment, and a connection with the world around me.

From a young age, I had always been drawn to animals. Their unconditional love and unwavering loyalty spoke to my heart in a way that nothing else could. It was during my teenage years that I received my first service dog, Spartan an instant, I felt a bond forming between us. Spartan understood me on a level that no human ever could. He saw beyond my physical appearance and connected with my spirit.

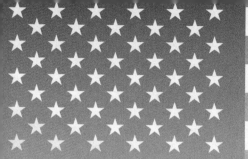

As he became my constant companion, I discovered a passion for training dogs in various sports and activities. Before I knew it, I was in the world of dock diving. Dock diving is a popular canine sport that showcases a dog's jumping and swimming abilities. It is a competition that tests the dog's agility, strength, and love for water. In dock diving, dogs leap from a raised platform or dock into a pool of water, aiming to achieve maximum distance or height.

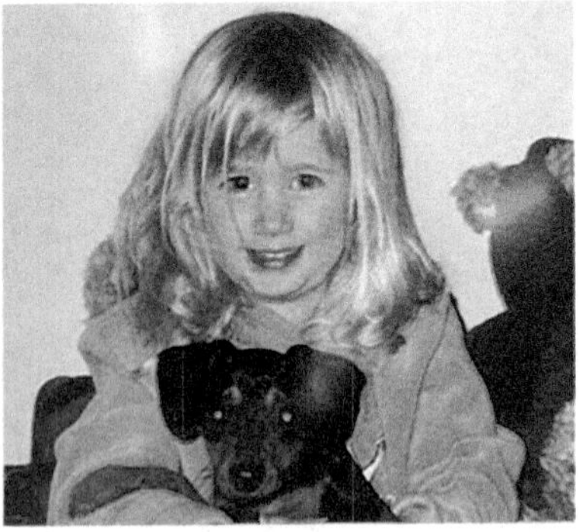

Jade Gronborg - with a girl's best friend

I began fostering dogs in need, offering them a temporary home filled with love and care. Each dog that entered my life brought with them a unique story of resilience and the capacity for growth. Witnessing their transformation from broken and fearful beings to confident and joyful companions was nothing short of awe-inspiring. The impact they had on my own healing journey was immeasurable.

Driven by a desire to make a difference not only in the lives of animals but also in the lives of people like me and my mother, Amy Rivera, I founded Jade Stone K9 Academy. It became a haven for dogs and humans, a place where we could rehabilitate and support one another through shared experiences. Just as my mother had dedicated her life to lymphedema, I wanted to provide a resource where animals could receive the rehabilitation they needed to thrive.

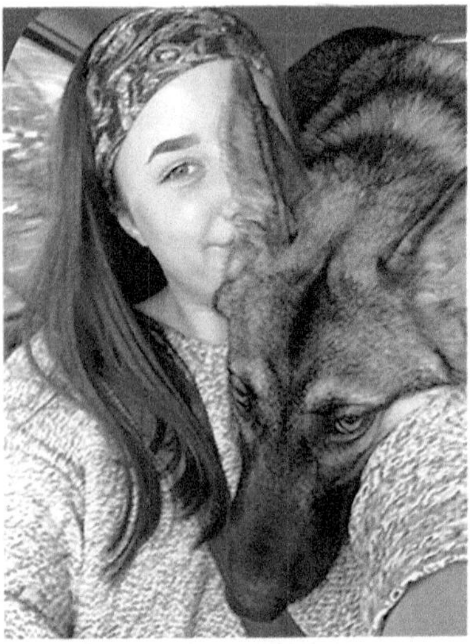

Jade Gronborg - Rest your head on my shoulder.

In my pursuit to understand the lymphatic system and its role in both human and animal health, I stumbled upon a fascinating revelation. Dogs, like humans, can develop lymphedema. It was a revelation that struck a chord deep

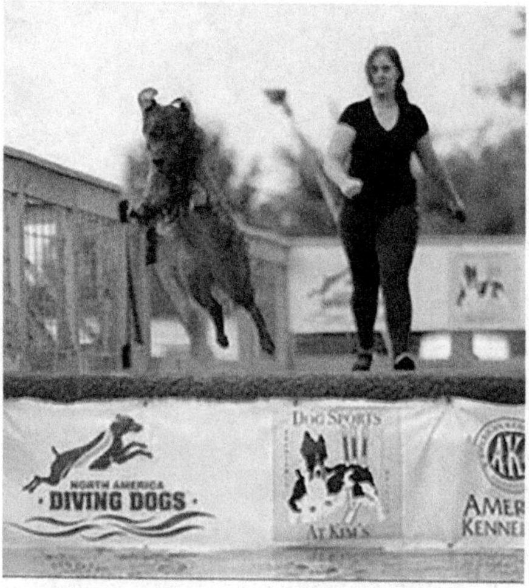

Jade Gronborg - Competing in Dock Diving

within me. I realized the importance of comprehending not only the challenges faced by humans with lymphedema but also the struggles that our beloved four-legged companions may encounter.

During one of our fostering experiences, a dog came into our care who had been born without a lymphatic system in his legs. It was a heartbreaking condition, yet it opened my eyes to the sheer resilience and adaptability of these remarkable animals. At that moment, I understood the profound connection between our experiences and the unbreakable bond we shared.

While having a role model as incredible as my mother has undoubtedly shaped my journey, it is important to acknowledge that not every day is easy. Living with lipedema comes with its own set of challenges, and I have faced additional medical issues directly related to my condition. Some days are harder than others, and there are moments when I question my own strength. But my mother has taught me a valuable lesson—to embrace my journey, to love my body, and, most importantly, to love myself.

For me, finding peace in the outdoors has been instrumental in my self-acceptance. I relish the freedom of exploring nature, whether it's bow fishing, swimming, working out, or simply spending time with fellow dog trainers who understand the deep connection we share with our canine companions.

Finding a place where you belong, especially when you feel out of place, is similar to the experience of a foster or lost animal. It's about discovering that sanctuary where you are embraced, understood, and valued for who you truly are. Just as every furry friend deserves a loving home, so do we yearn for that sense of belonging, where our hearts find solace and our spirits soar. Embrace your uniqueness, seek your pack, and together, create a haven where acceptance and love abound.

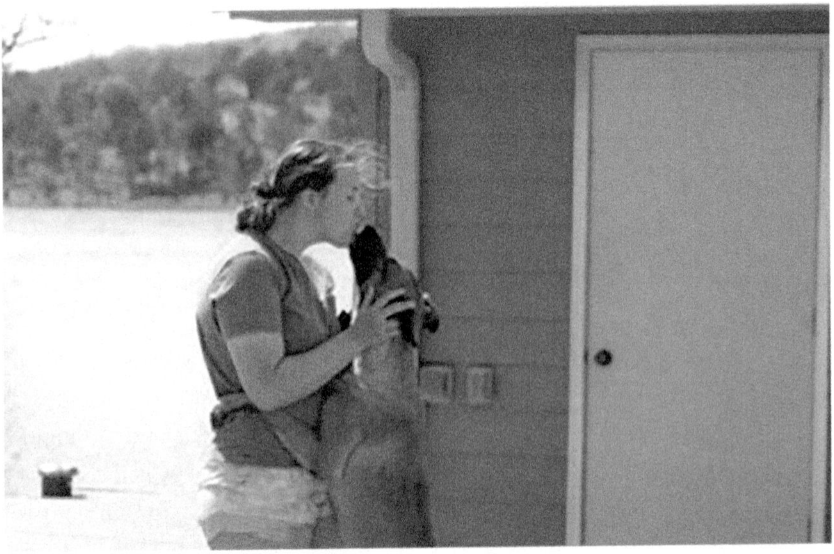

Jade Gronborg - Embracing the healing power of the canine-human bond

Dogs' companionship can bring immense comfort and support to those living with lymphedema and lipedema. Their unconditional love and intuitive nature can help alleviate stress and anxiety. Additionally, dogs can be trained to assist with daily activities such as fetching items or providing gentle pressure through their presence, offering practical assistance in managing lymphedema symptoms.

TOP TIP!

Embrace the healing power of the canine-human bond and consider the positive impact a furry friend can have on your journey.

AFTERWORD

We hope that you have found the stories, experiences and tip, both helpful and inspirational.

Living with lymphoedema isn't easy, as we know. It can be a full-time job, as we have read from some of our guests. However, it is just as important for us to try and find our *'new normal'* and live our lives with purpose.

If reading this book has inspired you to share your journey and provide tips to help others to live better with lymphoedema, please contact us. We hope to write more anthologies, with guests from all around the world, uniting the lymphoedema community.

Do get in touch.

Matt Hazledine *matt@lymphunited.com*

Amy Rivera *amy@winourfight.org*

PLEASE REMEMBER

Control your lymphoedema,
don't let your lymphoedema control you.

Stay Positive, Keep Talking, Make a Difference.

You are NOT alone!

MEET THE AUTHORS

Matt Hazledine

In 2011, at the age of 40, Matt experienced a severe episode of cellulitis in his left leg, which hospitalised him for 14 days. This subsequently caused a significant swelling called lymphoedema, a chronic lifelong disease with no cure.

During the initial years with lymphoedema, Matt really struggled to come to terms with adjusting his life to accommodate his very swollen leg. Through trial and error, he has worn every appropriate compression garment, tested almost every product, had all therapies known to him and two different types of surgery. He now knows what works for him and what doesn't.

In 2021, to commemorate 10 years of living with this life-changing condition, he wrote his first book 'How to Live Better with Lymphoedema – Meet the Experts' to share his extensive experiences and useful tips to help others and raise money for the Lymphoedema Research Fund. He is joined in the book by over 20 experts from the lymphoedema medical profession, each providing trusted information and guidance.

Matt also launched a patient-focused, one-stop-shop website for people with, or newly diagnosed with, lymphoedema. LymphoedemaUnited.com provides everything Matt would've wanted to know when he was diagnosed and hopes it saves time and stress for others going through a similar journey.

Over the past few years, he has been in a much happier and positive place and has continued his mission to help others living with the condition, whilst raising over £30,000 for various charities. Matt has been a Trustee of the Lymphoedema Support Network, featured in the Health Section of the Daily Mail, written for newsletters, blogs, podcasts and books, been interviewed on local hospital radio and public speaking at events, support groups and lymphoedema conferences.

He is a family man, who enjoys reading, playing golf, supporting Southend United and socialising with close friends. Matt is motivated to make a positive difference and help others to live better with lymphoedema.

If you would like to get in touch with Matt, please send him a message via his website *www.lymphoedemaunited.com* and follow him on Facebook, Instagram, YouTube and Twitter using @LymphUnited.

Amy Rivera

Amy Rivera, the founder of Ninjas Fighting Lymphedema Foundation, brings a wealth of personal experience and passion to the pages of this anthology. As a lymphedema warrior herself, Amy has faced the challenges and triumphs of living with this condition for over 30 years. Her relentless pursuit of knowledge, advocacy, and empowerment has not only transformed her own life but has inspired countless individuals around the world.

Through her unwavering determination, Amy has become a driving force in the lymphedema community, spreading awareness, providing support, and fostering a sense of belonging. Her journey, filled with misdiagnosis, failed procedures, and eventual healing, serves as a beacon of hope for others navigating their own lymphedema path.

In this anthology, Amy fearlessly shares her story, offering valuable insights, practical tips, and a message of resilience. Her contribution reflects her deep commitment to raising awareness, promoting education, and inspiring positive change. Amy's dedication to making a difference shines through her words, igniting a sense of empowerment and reminding us all that we are not alone in this journey.

Join us in celebrating Amy Rivera, a remarkable advocate, visionary, and warrior, as we dive into the profound and empowering stories that make up this transformative anthology.

ACKNOWLEDGEMENTS

Amy and Matt would like to take this opportunity to thank all our wonderfully inspiring guests, without whom this book would not have been created. May you all continue to live fulfilling and healthy lives and may our existing and new friendships flourish as foundations to build upon a united lymphoedema community. Thank you all.

Thank you also to Professor Christine Moffatt CBE, founder of the International Lymphoedema Framework (ILF), amongst many other incredible achievements. Your passion and purpose to bring healthcare to lymphoedema sufferers around the world, is selfless and life-changing for those you have helped.

With thanks to our publishing and design team at Wordzworth, Doug Morris and Kelly Roche for their professionalism, advice and for enabling this book to be assessable to the global lymphoedema community. Thank you.

DONATION TO CHARITIES

In the hope that this book is well-received and sells a few copies, Amy and Matt pledge to donate a proportion of annual pre-tax profits to many lymphoedema charities around the world, for many years to come. Dialogue has started with Professor Christine Moffatt CBE from the International Lymphoedema Framework, to see how the money raised can best be used to support the most needed places and help others to live better with lymphoedema.

Matt and Amy will keep you informed of future progress through their websites and social media.

Printed in Great Britain
by Amazon

31134150R10155